4.75

Understanding
Migraine
and Other Headaches

Dr Anne MacGregor

Published by Family Doctor Publications Limited
in association with the British Medical Association

616.857
MAC

© Family Doctor Publications 2002–2006
Updated 2004, 2005, 2006

Family Doctor Publications, PO Box 4664, Poole, Dorset BH15 1NN

ISBN: 1 903474 49 3

Contents

About the author

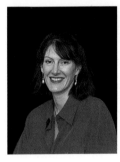 **Dr Anne MacGregor** is Director of Clinical Research at the City of London Migraine Clinic; she also works at St Bartholomew's Hospital, London. Her non-clinical work includes General Secretary of the International Headache Society and Medical Adviser to the Margaret Pyke Memorial Trust.

Introduction

What is a headache?

Fewer than two per cent of the population claim never to have had a headache. For most of the rest of us, headaches are fortunately infrequent and the cause is usually obvious, whether it is a hangover from too much alcohol, a deep pain over your eyes from a sinus infection or a throbbing pain in your cheek from a dental infection.

Other headaches may not have an obvious cause and, if they are frequent and severe, can cause significant concern and anxiety. Although doctors classify migraine and cluster headache (see pages 4–5) as benign (non-serious) conditions, they can seem very serious to the sufferer, who may be extremely disabled by attacks. It is not even just the attacks themselves that are disabling; fear of the next attack can affect a person's ability to lead a normal life.

What you'll find in this book

This book has been written to help anyone suffering from headaches to find ways to reduce the frequency and severity of the attacks and to lead a better quality of life. If you are prone to headaches, this book will help you understand what is triggering your symptoms and how you can combat them more successfully.

The central nervous system

The brain and spinal cord form the central nervous system (CNS). The brain performs many complex functions: for instance, it is the source of our consciousness, intelligence and creativity. It also monitors and controls, through the peripheral nervous system (PNS), most body processes – ranging from the automatic, such as breathing, to complex voluntary activities, such as riding a bicycle.

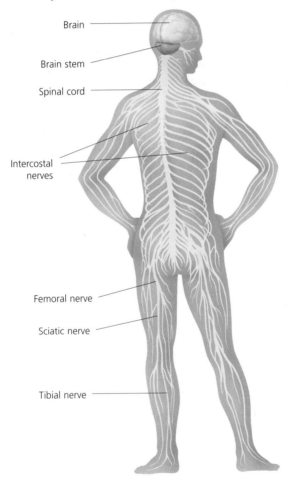

Brain

Brain stem

Spinal cord

Intercostal
nerves

Femoral nerve

Sciatic nerve

Tibial nerve

There are chapters on migraine triggers and living with migraine, as well as on other types of headaches, such as chronic daily headaches. The chapters on headaches in women, children and elderly people highlight common causes of headaches in these specific groups of people and provide some possible self-help measures to ease the symptoms.

This book is not intended to help you diagnose the cause of your headaches yourself. Information in this book cannot replace the advice of a doctor or medical specialist, who will be able to confirm the suspected diagnosis and offer advice suitable for your individual case.

Certainly, if the nature of your headaches is uncertain, if the attacks become more frequent or severe or if your symptoms change in any way, you must seek medical advice immediately. Severe headaches are rarely the result of anything sinister, such as a brain tumour or stroke. However, these causes must be ruled out before the more likely explanation, such as migraine, can be confirmed.

Recognising your headache

Each headache has its own particular pattern of symptoms. The table on the next two pages shows the usual pattern of symptoms of some of the more common types of headaches. As there are no diagnostic tests for most of the common types of headaches, listening to the story told by the patient is usually the only way in which a doctor can make a diagnosis of the type of headaches. These non-migraine headaches are discussed in more detail in later chapters.

Characteristics of the more

Characteristic	Migraine	Muscle contraction headache
Age at onset of headaches	Childhood/teens/20s	Any age but rarely children
Frequency with which headaches occur	Episodic: average one to two attacks per month but very variable	Episodic or daily
Duration of headaches	Part of a day up to three days	Hours to weeks
Principal symptoms	Often unilateral	Localised
	Severe	Tender to touch
	Throbbing	
Associated symptoms	Nausea	Tender neck/shoulder muscles
	Vomiting	
	Photophobia (dislike of bright light)	
	General malaise (feeling unwell)	
Mood during headaches	Usually normal but can be associated with depression	Normal
General health	Well	Well
How often is medication taken to treat symptoms?	Episodic	Episodic
Effect of medication	Right medication usually gives relief	Response in 20 to 30 minutes

common types of headaches

Stress/depression headache	Chronic daily headaches	Cluster headache (rare)
Any age	30s/40s	30s
Usually daily	Daily	Episodic: average of one to two attacks per day for six weeks Chronic: average of one to two attacks per day
Continuous	Continuous	Half-an-hour to two hours
All-over pressure	All over	Unilateral, centring on one eye
Band around your head	Diffuse and dull	
Weight on your head	May have additional migraine attacks	
Mild	Mild unless additional migraine attacks	Affected side: eye and nose water Affected side: eye reddens
Depressed	Flat/'suppressed'	Normal
General malaise (feeling unwell)	General malaise (feeling unwell)	Normal but often smokes or history of smoking
Frequent, often daily	None or daily, particularly if associated with overuse of acute medication	Episodic
Minimal response	Minimal response	Right medication usually gives relief

KEY POINTS

- Severe headaches are rarely the result of anything sinister

- Each headache has its own particular pattern of symptoms

Different types of migraine

What is migraine?

The name 'migraine' is derived from the word 'he**micran**ia' meaning a one-sided headache, although the migraine headache can be generalised. Migraine headache is often described as a throbbing pain that gets worse on physical activity. Although the pain may be severe, migraine is not in itself life threatening, although a bad attack often feels like it.

What are the symptoms?

Migraine is, however, more than just a headache and the headache is not necessarily the major symptom. Some attacks are preceded by visual disturbances. Other typical symptoms include nausea, vomiting, and sensitivity to light, noise and smell. Many sufferers cannot bear even the thought of food, whereas others find that eating takes the edge off their nausea.

Migraine has been likened to a power cut. During a migraine, you may find that your whole body seems to shut down for a while, and you want to hide away until the attack is over.

Do you have migraine?

Ask yourself the following questions – try to be as honest with yourself as you can:

- Do you have headaches that last between 4 and 72 hours?
- Is the pain usually one-sided and/or throbbing?
- Do you feel sick or vomit with the headaches?
- Does light or noise bother you when you have a headache?
- Do you find it difficult to concentrate when you have a headache and sometimes have to stop and sit or lie down?
- Is your general health good between these attacks?

If you answer 'yes' to most of these questions, you probably have migraine.

Lethargy (a lack of energy) is a common symptom and every task may seem to take twice as long – if it is possible to tackle it at all. Your stomach may stop working normally, making it harder for medication to be absorbed into your bloodstream, especially if treatment is delayed.

Many people have to lie still in a quiet, darkened room until the attack is over. If medication doesn't control an attack, you may find that your symptoms improve after a good sleep. Other people find that vomiting will relieve their symptoms. Migraine lasts anything from four hours to three days, with complete freedom from symptoms between attacks.

Who gets migraine?

At a conservative estimate, migraine affects about 10 to 12 per cent of the population at some time in their lives. In the UK, this amounts to over six million people. It is difficult to give a precise figure because some people may have only three or four attacks in a lifetime and not recognise them as migraine.

Gender

Migraine affects more women than men in a ratio of about three to one. Hormonal changes in women are the obvious reason for this difference between the sexes and account for the fact that, until puberty, migraine is equally prevalent in boys and girls.

In one large survey, researchers found that, of those questioned, 8 per cent of men and 25 per cent of women had had a headache with features of migraine at some time in their lives.

Age

At least 90 per cent of people who get migraine have their first attack before the age of 40. For most people, migraine starts during their teens or early 20s, although it has been diagnosed in young children and even babies. It is rare for anyone over the age of 50 to experience their first attack of migraine, although migraine can return at this time of life after years of respite.

Even though migraine starts when you are young, it is often not a problem until later life when attacks become more frequent. Studies show that women are most likely to have problems with migraine, particularly in their 30s and 40s. In men, the pattern is fairly consistent throughout their lives. Migraine usually improves in midlife for both sexes, although an unfortunate few do continue to have attacks.

What are the different types of migraine?

The two most frequently encountered types of migraine differ only in the presence or absence of an 'aura'. An aura is a group of neurological symptoms that precede the headache, most often visual (see below).

About 70 to 80 per cent of migraineurs (people who suffer from migraine) experience attacks of migraine without aura (formerly known as common migraine); 10 per cent have migraine with aura (formerly known as classic migraine); 15 to 20 per cent have both types of attacks. Less than one per cent of attacks are of aura alone with no headache developing. Other types of migraine are extremely rare (see page 18).

The five phases of migraine

Migraine is more than just a headache. You may feel that your body has had a power cut – it shuts down for a while and you want to hide away. During an attack, you may experience a heightened sensitivity to light, sound and smell, not want to eat, experience nausea or vomiting, have an inability to concentrate and feel generally extremely unwell. These other symptoms may cause you more distress than the headache itself. In fact, migraine can be divided into five distinct phases:

1 premonitory (warning signs)

2 aura

3 headache

4 resolution

5 postdromal (recovery).

Premonitory phase

Two-thirds of migraineurs experience these warning symptoms, although you may not recognise them for what they are until you become accustomed to them and know what to look for. These symptoms include very subtle changes in your mood or behaviour, which may be more apparent to your friends and family than they are to you. They include:

- Mood changes: irritability, feeling 'high' or 'low'.

- Behavioural changes: hyperactive, obsessional, clumsy, lethargic.

- Neurological symptoms: tired or yawning, difficulty finding the right words, dislike of light and sound, difficulty in focusing your eyes.

- Muscular symptoms: generalised aches and pains.

- Gut symptoms: nausea, craving for certain foods (often sweet), not wanting to eat, constipation or diarrhoea.

- Changes in fluid balance: thirst, wanting to pass water more often or fluid retention.

These symptoms are sometimes blamed as triggers for the attack. For example, if you crave chocolate, eat it and then wake up the next morning with a migraine, it wasn't necessarily the chocolate that caused the migraine. It is much more likely that the craving was a symptom of an attack that had already started. Premonitory symptoms usually begin subtly and develop over a period of up to 24 hours before the headache starts.

Aura

Many people, including some doctors, mistakenly think that it can't be migraine unless an aura occurs. But only 20 to 30 per cent of all migraine attacks are accompanied by an aura. Of those people who do have attacks with aura, most also have attacks without aura.

The headaches are similar regardless of whether or not they followed an aura. However, many sufferers are not aware that the headaches that they have without the aura are still migraine.

Aura can affect vision and, less commonly, sensation or speech. When several aura symptoms are present, they usually follow each other in succession. There may or may not be a gap of anything up to an hour between the end of the aura and the onset of the headache. Most people say they feel a bit 'spaced out' during this gap.

Visual disturbances are the most common aura symptoms and can take several forms, a typical description being:

'... bright zigzag lines and I lose part of my vision during this time, all prior to the head pain. It lasts anything from 20 to 45 minutes. Then my vision restores itself at the same time as the head pain starts.'

Other visual symptoms
These include:

- Blind spots – varying from part of a letter missing on a page, looking like a misprint, to somebody's chin missing or the absence of half your field of vision – culminating in pulsating lines around objects.

- Impression of the scene being viewed though a shattered mirror.

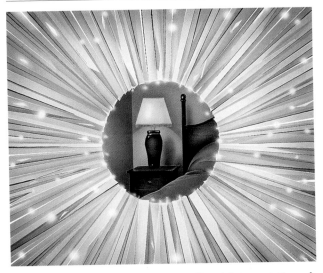

This illustration shows a migraine sufferer's interpretation of what is seen in the aura stage of the migraine attack. The aura precedes the onset of the headache.

- Difficulty in focusing – seeming to see what is below what you are actually looking at.

- Flashing lights.

The zigzag lines described in the first account are known as *fortification spectra* (because of their similarity to the plan of a mediaeval castle) and usually start as a small dot in your visual field, which gradually enlarges and becomes surrounded by a shimmering edge of zigzags, leaving a small blind spot in its wake (*scintillating scotoma*).

The aura stage usually takes about 5 to 60 minutes from start to finish. The symptoms affect both your eyes, although they may often seem to affect one eye only. If you close or cover the eye that seems to be affected, you will notice that they are present in the other eye as well.

Disturbances of other sensations are less common. These nearly always occur together with visual symptoms and are rarely the only symptom of aura. Typical disturbances of sensation include pins and needles starting in the fingers of one hand, which spread up your arm to affect one side of your face or tongue. It is unusual for these symptoms to affect your legs.

Dysphasia, meaning difficulty in finding the right words, can start as an aura but can occur throughout the migraine. One sufferer describes this as 'loss of memory of words – any words – inability to put sentences together or to distinguish between letters and numbers'.

Headache

This phase can last for anything up to three days. The headache is often one-sided and throbbing but can affect both sides of your head. It can occur on the same or opposite side to the aura, if aura has occurred. Movement makes the headache worse and, if it is severe, you may need to lie down or sit still. However, the headache is only one symptom of this phase of migraine. One sufferer describes it as follows:

'The head pain lasts about 18 hours. My head throbs and feels like I've got a drill boring through my brain. Sometimes it pounds so much that I'm terrified my head is going to explode, even though I know that it can't. My neck and shoulder muscles are really tender and I can't bear to comb my hair. Even normal lights hurt my eyes and I feel nauseous, although I'm not as sick as I used to be in the past. I usually feel very cold at the beginning of an attack and then later on I become very hot. I also become very irritable and depressed.'

The most common accompanying symptoms during this headache phase are nausea, vomiting, and sensitivity to light, sound and smell. Although some people can't stand the thought of eating anything without feeling even more sick, others find that eating helps, particularly starchy foods such as bread or pasta.

Sometimes the accompanying symptoms are more troublesome and distressing than the headache itself. For example, one patient describes a feeling of 'total confusion and disorientation – the most distressing part of the migraine attacks I have'. For others, continued nausea and repeated vomiting are the worst features of migraine.

Resolution

There is great variability in the way the attack comes to an end. You may notice, for example, that if you can control your symptoms enough to be able to get some sleep, you'll wake up feeling much better. However, this restorative property of sleep doesn't happen in everyone.

Children often find that they feel much better after they have been sick – often with seemingly miraculous results. For others, attacks improve with effective medication. A few find that nothing really works and the attack has to burn itself out.

Recovery (postdromal)

After the headache has gone, you may feel drained and washed out for another 24 hours or so. Some people describe this as feeling like they've 'been wrung through a mangle'. Others feel very energetic and even euphoric.

Between migraine attacks

If a sufferer's only problem is a migraine, the typical response to the question 'How do you feel between attacks?' is 'Fine'. If, however, your symptoms continue between attacks, or if you have other medical problems, it is important to speak to your doctor so that he or she can try to find their cause.

Frequency of attacks

Migraine is not a static condition. The frequency of attacks can vary considerably in the same person over time. You may have attacks that come once or twice a month during a bad patch, whereas a few unlucky people may have a spell of attacks occurring once a week. This could be followed by a gap of several months, or even years, without an attack, often for no apparent reason.

One important point to note is that true migraine does not occur daily. It seems that, after an attack of a full-blown migraine, there is a period of a few days during which, whatever you do, you can't trigger an attack. However, migraine sufferers can get other kinds of headache too, some of which occur daily.

Although these daily symptoms are usually not severe, migraine often increases in frequency or severity, making it difficult for the sufferer to cope.

How migraine changes over time

Children typically have short and sharp attacks lasting for only a few hours. With increasing age, the attacks tend to last longer but are less severe. In adult life, their frequency varies considerably over time, many people experiencing periods of respite that can last for several years, coupled with other times when migraine attacks can be quite frequent.

It is not just the frequency and duration of attacks that change over time; your symptoms can also change. You can change from suffering mostly attacks of migraine with aura to migraine without aura and vice versa. An aura is often apparent in childhood, but it may disappear for many years only to return in later life, unaccompanied by a headache.

Hormonal changes, such as those that occur in pregnancy or with the use of oral contraceptives or hormone replacement therapy (HRT), have an extremely variable effect on migraine. In some people, this effect is beneficial. For others, however, migraine without aura can convert to migraine with aura and the frequency and severity of attacks may worsen. When the hormonal levels return to normal after a pregnancy, or when you discontinue the oral contraceptive pill or HRT, migraine often reverts back to the previous type, although the frequency of attack may remain more severe.

Fears

An attack of migraine can be very frightening. If you experience visual disturbances, you may be scared that you will permanently lose your vision.

Many people are afraid that their migraine is a symptom of a stroke or brain tumour. Fortunately, these worrying causes are rare, and you would usually be aware of other symptoms such as unsteadiness or weakness in a limb rather than headache.

Although the symptoms of migraine can be disturbing, they are not life threatening and your body returns to normal between attacks. Between attacks, most migraineurs feel their usual selves – forgetting how bad they felt with the migraine until another attack starts. For others, fear of the next attack can lead to social isolation and even an inability to work.

Other types of migraine
Migraine aura without headache
If you have attacks of migraine with aura for many years, you may find that the headache becomes less severe with time or doesn't occur at all. These attacks are then called 'migraine aura without headache'. It is rare for attacks to have always occurred without a headache. If you are over 50 and have never had a migraine but develop 'aura' for the first time, consult your doctor. Other medical causes that give rise to similar symptoms must be ruled out.

Status migrainosus
This term is used to describe attacks of migraine that may last for longer than the generally accepted 72 hours. Sometimes, this can be the result of a muscle-contraction headache (see page 125) developing from pain and tenderness in your neck and shoulder muscles caused by the migraine.

Status migrainosus can be recognised when the usual symptoms of nausea and sensitivity to light resolve after a couple of days but the headache persists. Anti-inflammatory drugs, such as aspirin or ibuprofen, usually ease the symptoms but if they persist you should see your doctor.

A few people taking specific treatments such as 'triptans' (see page 63) find that their migraine is effectively treated on the first day, but the attack comes back again the next day. Treatment with a second dose of the triptan is effective, although the same pattern can occur for several days. This is more common in people whose migraine attacks usually last for two or three days, and most common in women with an attack around the time of menstruation.

Rare types of migraine

There are several other types that are considered to be variants of migraine, but the link of some of these with migraine is controversial and all are extremely rare. In addition, the terms are often incorrectly used, so it is important to have the diagnosis confirmed by a doctor or medical specialist. Rare types of migraine include: basilar type, hemiplegic, ophthalmoplegic, retinal and migrainous infarction.

Basilar-type migraine

The symptoms of basilar-type migraine are controlled from a part of the brain known as the brain stem. These symptoms include difficulty in articulating words, vertigo (an illusion that the environment is constantly moving), ringing in the ears, double vision and unsteadiness, in addition to the more common aura symptoms. Severe attacks may result in fainting and even a sudden loss of consciousness, which can be very frightening. These symptoms last up to 60 minutes and are followed by a typical migraine headache.

However, similar symptoms can occur when anxiety or fear of a migraine results in attacks of overbreathing, called hyperventilation. These symptoms resolve by breathing gently in and out of a paper bag, which restores the balance of oxygen and carbon dioxide in the body.

Hemiplegic migraine

In this type of migraine, attacks of migraine with aura are associated with weakness or paralysis of the whole of one side of the body, affecting both the arm and leg. This persists throughout the attack, sometimes for several days, until the headache subsides. In subsequent attacks, the opposite side may be affected. When there is a family history of identical attacks, it is called familial hemiplegic migraine.

Ophthalmoplegic migraine

This condition is extremely rare. The headache is associated with one-sided paralysis of one or more of the nerves that control the eye muscles responsible for eye movement.

Although these symptoms must be investigated, no underlying cause is found if they are the result of migraine. The paralysis may affect one side in one attack and the other side in another attack. Attacks usually occur very infrequently, with several months between episodes.

Retinal migraine

These are attacks of blind spots (see page 12) that affect vision in one eye only and are associated with a headache. If the eye is examined with an ophthalmoscope (an instrument for looking inside the eye), it is normal between attacks and during them.

Migrainous infarction

An infarct is the death of tissue as a result of an inadequate blood supply. Symptoms ranging from permanent blind spots in one eye to a full stroke (see 'Fears', page 17) have been reported after attacks of migraine, but these are extremely rare.

It is difficult to establish a direct link because other causes of these events can coexist with migraine. A diagnosis of migrainous infarction would be considered only if the infarct occurs during the course of a typical migraine attack rather than at any other time.

What happens to your brain and body during a migraine?
Why do some people get migraine and others don't?

People who have frequent migraines are thought to have 'hyperexcitable' brains, meaning that they are much more sensitive to stimuli that would not affect someone not prone to migraine. This sensitivity is perhaps in part genetically determined, influencing the threshold for triggering attacks.

What happens in the brain during a migraine?

For centuries, it was believed that migraine aura was caused by the constriction of blood vessels in the part of the brain at the back of the head responsible for processing vision, known as the visual cortex. The headache was thought to result from subsequent swelling of blood vessels in the brain.

More recently, the underlying events have become better understood. Changes in the blood vessels are now thought to be secondary to more important changes in brain chemistry.

One chemical that is released within the brain is serotonin, also known by its chemical name 5-hydroxytryptamine or 5HT. It is thought to play a major role in the migraine process because it has a powerful effect on the size of the blood vessels. It also promotes blood clotting by causing platelets (blood cell fragments) to stick together.

Ninety per cent of serotonin is concentrated in the gut, where it helps control the secretion of digestive fluids and the muscular movements of the intestines. Between two and eight per cent is found in the brain.

Different areas of the brain have specific functions

It was believed that migraine aura was caused by the constriction of blood vessels in the visual cortex at the back of the brain.

Premotor cortex coordinates complex movements such as playing a musical instrument

Motor cortex sends signals to muscles to cause voluntary movements

Primary sensory cortex receives data about sensations in the skin, muscles, joints and organs

Prefrontal cortex deals with behaviour and personality

Sensory association cortex analyses data about sensations

Visual association cortex forms images once visual data have been analysed

Broca's area is involved in the formation of speech

Primary auditory cortex distinguishes the particular qualities of sound

Auditory association cortex analyses and interprets sound data

Primary visual cortex receives nerve impulses from the eye

Wernicke's area interprets written and spoken language

Premonitory symptoms

Triggers such as stress, bright lights, menstruation, dehydration or other factors appear to activate specific centres in the brain stem, the area at the base of the brain, close to the spinal cord. These cause brain chemicals such as serotonin to rise, disrupting the normal function of the hypothalamus. This organ in the brain is likely to be responsible for premonitory signs and symptoms of migraine, such as mood changes, food cravings, drowsiness, thirst and yawning. These signs and symptoms may occur several hours, or even as long as a day or so, before the headache pain begins.

Migraine aura
It has been suggested that constriction of blood vessels within the brain triggers further changes in brain activity known as cortical spreading depression (CSD). This is a wave of electrical activity that moves across the surface of the brain at a rate of about three millimetres per minute, similar to the rate at which the visual aura develops. Hence CSD is thought to be associated with migraine aura.

Migraine headache
The headache of migraine is thought to result from swelling of the blood vessels on the outside of the brain, called the meningeal arteries. The swollen blood vessels release inflammatory agents known as neuropeptides, irritating the nerves surrounding them. This activates the nerves, which send pain signals to the trigeminal ganglion, located just above the roof of the mouth.

The trigeminal ganglion contains a dense cluster of nerve cells of the trigeminal nerve. It receives signals about conditions inside the skull, delivering sensory stimuli to the brain from the face, teeth and tongue.

When activated, the trigeminal nerve also transmits pain impulses to the trigeminal nucleus caudalis in the brain stem, which relays pain impulses to the thalamus. The thalamus, deep within the brain stem, is a routing station for the incoming sensory impulses of sight, sound, taste and touch.

Changes in blood flow in the brain may cause migraine

There is still controversy about the precise cause of migraine attacks and their effects on the brain. During an attack, arteries in the head first constrict (narrow) then dilate (widen), causing a disturbance in the blood flow to the brain.

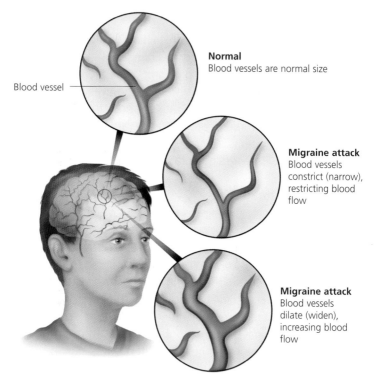

Blood vessel

Normal
Blood vessels are normal size

Migraine attack
Blood vessels constrict (narrow), restricting blood flow

Migraine attack
Blood vessels dilate (widen), increasing blood flow

Incoming sensory stimuli are processed to produce the appropriate physical reactions and emotions. Information from the thalamus passes up to the cerebral cortex, the outermost part of the brain, which decodes the messages into our experience of pain. These pain pathways are thought to contribute to the

How nerve cells transmit messages

Essentially, your brain is like a bundle of telephone wires transmitting and receiving messages within your brain and to and from other parts of your body. Some of the messages are sent by electrical impulses; others depend on the release and transmission of particular chemicals called neurotransmitters.

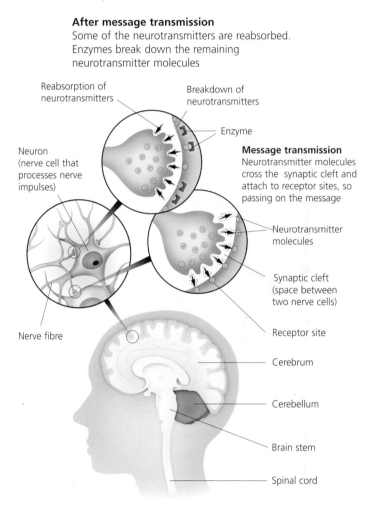

After message transmission
Some of the neurotransmitters are reabsorbed. Enzymes break down the remaining neurotransmitter molecules

Reabsorption of neurotransmitters

Breakdown of neurotransmitters

Enzyme

Neuron (nerve cell that processes nerve impulses)

Message transmission
Neurotransmitter molecules cross the synaptic cleft and attach to receptor sites, so passing on the message

Neurotransmitter molecules

Synaptic cleft (space between two nerve cells)

Nerve fibre

Receptor site

Cerebrum

Cerebellum

Brain stem

Spinal cord

worsening of migraine pain, as well as the associated symptoms of nausea and light and sound sensitivity. Eventually, brain chemicals and blood vessels return to normal and the attack ends.

The role of serotonin in migraine headache

Studies have shown that attacks can be provoked by an injection of reserpine, a drug that releases serotonin from body stores, inducing migraine headaches just in susceptible individuals. Further evidence that serotonin is implicated in migraine is that an intravenous infusion of serotonin itself, given during an attack of migraine, can relieve symptoms, although the precise mechanism of this action is still unclear. Unfortunately, its use as a treatment is limited by side effects, such as shortness of breath, nausea and generalised constriction of blood vessels, resulting in faintness, tingling and numbness.

Recent research has shown that targeting drugs to affect specific actions of serotonin can treat the symptoms of migraine with few unwanted effects. These drugs, known as triptans, are available on prescription from a doctor (see page 63).

KEY POINTS

- A migraine is more than just a bad headache, and headache is not necessarily the major symptom

- Migraine affects more women than men, possibly as a result of hormonal differences

- Most people have migraine without aura, some have migraine with aura and some have both types

- An aura may include disturbances in vision, sensation and speech

- Migraine can be divided into five distinct phases: premonitory (warning) signs, aura, headache, resolution and recovery

- Migraine seems to be caused by changes in certain brain chemicals, especially serotonin

Migraine triggers

Many and varied

There is no single trigger for a migraine attack. In a study at the City of London Migraine Clinic, 79 per cent of the patients questioned were aware of precipitating factors, the most common being stress, hormones, tiredness and missing meals. Most patients noted that several precipitating factors acting together were necessary to trigger an attack.

The migraine 'threshold'

Imagine a migraine 'threshold' that is determined by your genetic makeup. This threshold is also raised or lowered by external factors, as well as internal changes in your brain. Varying triggers occur over a period of time. If a sufficient number of different internal and environmental triggers build up to cross the current threshold, a migraine attack is initiated.

This explains why you do not always get a migraine attack in similar situations – perhaps your threshold fluctuates or the number or importance of triggers varies. Consequently, missing a meal and less obvious triggers, such as flickering sunlight or a lack of sleep, do not always bring on an attack. However, if any or all of these are combined with a period of stress at work or hormone changes, an attack may occur.

The typical pattern of a migraine attack

Migraine sufferers have a 'threshold' that is determined by their genetic makeup (internal factors). This threshold can also be raised or lowered by external factors such as stress. If a sufficient number of internal and external triggers build up, the threshold may be crossed and a migraine attack initiated.

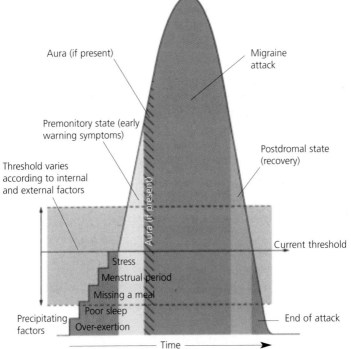

Aura (if present)

Migraine attack

Premonitory state (early warning symptoms)

Postdromal state (recovery)

Threshold varies according to internal and external factors

Aura (if present)

Current threshold

Stress
Menstrual period
Missing a meal
Poor sleep
Over-exertion

Precipitating factors

End of attack

Time

Drugs taken daily to prevent migraine may work by raising your threshold, so more triggers are necessary before an attack is triggered.

Migraine triggers

The triggers for migraine are many and varied, but are the same as those that provoke 'normal' headaches in apparently non-migrainous people. The triggers are not the same for everyone, and not necessarily the same for different attacks in the same person.

However, some triggers are more important than others. The most common trigger, particularly in children, is hunger or eating too little. In women, hormonal fluctuations associated with the menstrual cycle can provoke migraine.

In some cases, it may be difficult to distinguish triggers from premonitory (warning) symptoms. For example, if you are sensitive to light in the hours before the headache starts, you will be more aware of sunlight flickering through the trees while driving. Similarly, premonitory carbohydrate cravings may provoke a desire for chocolate, which is then incorrectly blamed as the cause of an attack.

In both cases, you should consider these symptoms to be a warning of the attack. The symptoms should prompt you to act to prevent the ensuing attack, either by early treatment where appropriate or more usually by dealing with any identified triggers.

Insufficient food

Delayed or missed meals often result in a slight fall in the individual's blood sugar, thus triggering migraine. This is usually the most important trigger in children, particularly when they are going through a growth spurt or are involved in strenuous exercise. It explains why many children come home from school with a bad headache – they just haven't eaten sufficient food often enough to maintain their blood sugar level.

Insufficient food may also be an important migraine trigger in adults. Missing breakfast typically triggers attacks in the late morning, whereas missing lunch may trigger attacks in the late afternoon. If attacks are present when you wake up, it is worthwhile reconsidering the time that you eat your evening meal – which may be quite early. A bowl of cereal last thing at night might be all you need to treat your migraine.

Many migraineurs find that they need to eat frequent snacks, every four hours or so, to avoid the fluctuations in blood sugar that may act as a trigger. Sugary snacks and chocolate are fine to eat – but best at the end of a meal and not in place of one.

Dehydration is a common cause of headache and is also implicated in migraine. A recent study of increasing daily fluid intake by at least one litre per day showed that increased water intake reduced the total number of hours and intensity of headache episodes.

Food allergy

Allergy, usually in relation to certain foods, is often considered to be an important trigger for migraine but it remains a highly contentious subject. Many foods have been implicated in migraine, ranging from cheese, chocolate, citrus fruits, to pickled foods (such as herrings) and even Chinese food. Although there is no doubt that certain foods can trigger attacks of migraine in susceptible people, in most such cases the link between eating the suspect food(s) and the onset of migraine is so obvious that the person quickly learns to avoid the food.

The most frequently cited trigger is alcohol. Certain types of alcohol contain chemicals (called congeners) that can either directly affect blood vessels or provoke the release of other chemicals thought to be involved in migraine. The migraineur is sensitive to certain components of the alcoholic drink. Certain red wines contain more of these potent chemicals and are therefore more likely to trigger an attack than purer drinks such as vodka. This type of response is not a true allergic reaction.

Trigger factors that can precipitate a migraine attack

This chart shows the most common migraine trigger factors. Not all apply to every attack and usually more than one factor is involved.

Dietary

- Missing meals
- Delayed meals
- Inadequate quantity
- Caffeine withdrawal
- Dehydration
- Specific foods are rare but will be obvious (see 'Food allergy', page 31)

Environmental triggers

- Bright or flickering lights
- Over-exertion/exercise
- Travel
- Weather changes
- Strong smells

Hormonal changes in women

- Menstruation
- Oral contraception
- Pregnancy (may exacerbate focal symptoms but usually migraine improves in second and third trimester)
- Menopause
- Hormone replacement therapy (HRT)

Trigger factors that can precipitate a migraine attack (contd)

Illness
For example, viral infection such as a cold or flu

Sleep
- Oversleeping – lying in
- Lack of sleep

Emotional triggers
For example, argument, excitement, stress

Head and neck pains
- Eyes, sinuses, neck, teeth or jaw pain

A true allergic response is when an antigen (the substance triggering an allergy, in this case a suspect food) triggers the production of specific antibodies, which can be measured in the bloodstream. Despite intense research, no specific antigen–antibody reaction has been identified in migraineurs as a result of eating trigger foods, so the term 'food sensitivity' or 'food intolerance' has been favoured.

It is therefore unlikely that allergy testing is worthwhile in migraine except in a very small number of cases. Unfortunately, many unqualified practitioners have offered unscientific tests. These have led many migraineurs to follow strict diets that may themselves cause migraine, as a result of nutritional deficiencies, if they are continued for long periods of time.

Several research groups have carefully tested controlled elimination diets in which all but a few simple foods are excluded from the diet and then gradually other foods are introduced one by one. Some people did very well on these diets but they were so restrictive that many people could not maintain them. In one study, 40 per cent of patients had dropped out within the first 6 weeks and by the end of the study only 10 per cent found that their symptoms had improved.

Whatever the link between food and migraine, too many people strictly avoid suspect foods without first discovering whether or not these foods contribute to their own headaches. If you think that a certain food is triggering your attacks, you should eliminate that food from your diet for several weeks, keeping a diary to see if there is any change in your attacks. If not, you can reinstate the food and avoid another suspect food. Stricter elimination diets should be done only under the supervision of a doctor or dietitian.

Dietary control can be socially disabling – it is very difficult to avoid the chocolate mousse or French cheeses served with delicious wines at a dinner party. In addition, the fear of the effects of the food may in itself be sufficient to trigger an attack.

Many migraineurs can control their attacks with minimal food avoidance by eating regularly, in addition to identifying and avoiding non-dietary triggers. Only if these measures are ineffective is it worthwhile seeking the advice of a qualified allergy specialist. Ask your doctor to refer you.

Exercise

If you are unfit, strenuous exercise is likely to trigger a migraine as well as muscle aches and pains. This puts many people off taking exercise when, in fact, regular exercise can help prevent migraine attacks. Fit people have improved blood sugar balance, better breathing and better pain control compared with unfit people – exercise stimulates your body to release natural pain-controlling chemicals called endorphins and enkephalins, relieves depression and promotes a general sense of well-being.

You should start a new exercise programme gently, building up the pace gradually over several weeks. It is important to keep the exercise sessions regular. Short frequent sessions are more beneficial than long infrequent sessions – the latter sometimes doing more harm than good.

You should be aware that exercise can change your fluid and blood sugar levels and that dehydration and a low blood sugar can be potent migraine triggers. Children appear to be particularly susceptible to the effects of strenuous exercise, developing migraine after a hard game of football. In many cases, drinking lots of fluids and sucking glucose tablets before and during exercise can prevent these attacks.

Occasionally, migraine can be triggered by a blow to the head during exercise. A doctor should check this out, because, in a few cases, the migraine-like symptoms can be associated with injury to the brain.

Hormones

In a study at the City of London Migraine Clinic, more than 50 per cent of women reported that they were more likely to have a migraine attack around the time of their menstrual period. Although most women also have attacks at other times of their menstrual cycle, a small percentage only have attacks that are exclusively associated with their periods. These attacks can usually be controlled with standard migraine management strategies; a few women with obvious hormonal triggers may benefit from specific intervention as described in 'Headaches in women' (see page 90).

Other hormonal changes, such as the use of hormonal contraception, can exacerbate migraine in some women and improve it in others. The years leading up to the menopause are typically associated with an increased frequency of migraine, particularly menstrual migraine. The hormonal fluctuations associated with a worsening of migraine at this time can be controlled using hormone replacement therapy, which may be suggested anyway if other menopausal symptoms, such as hot flushes and night sweats, are present.

Illness

Most people will get a headache when they have a cold or viral infection, but migraine can also occur during this time. It is uncertain whether the illness itself is a trigger or if being ill lowers your attack threshold so that fewer triggers can produce an attack.

If you're coming down with a cold, stock up with migraine treatments as well as cold remedies. Make sure, however, that you don't take more than the recommended dose of your chosen painkiller and remember that many cold remedies also contain painkillers.

Sleep

The true association between migraine and sleep is poorly understood. Migraine is often present on waking. A lack of sleep is recognised as a trigger for migraine. Conversely, sleeping during an attack may resolve your symptoms.

Other factors may also be important. For example, a lack of sleep can result from depression, anxiety, menopausal hot flushes, or delayed bedtime as a result of social events, work or study. Each of these could be a migraine trigger.

Many people notice that sleeping in for even just half an hour longer than usual, or lying in bed dozing, can result in migraine. This may be one cause of weekend migraine.

What is clear is that, if you suffer from migraine, you should try to stick to a fixed sleep pattern, going to bed at night and getting up in the morning at regular times. Shift workers should try to avoid frequent changes of shift times, where possible.

Stress

Anxiety and emotion play an important role in headache and migraine. Most migraineurs have found that they cope with stress without having more migraine attacks at the time, but have attacks when they relax. Stress rarely occurs without a knock-on effect on other migraine triggers, often resulting in missed meals, poor sleep and increased muscle tension.

Although stress is often unavoidable, it is important to try to reduce the effects of other triggers by eating regularly and getting adequate sleep. This can also help you cope with the stress more efficiently.

Musculoskeletal pain

In a study at the City of London Migraine Clinic, neck pain was a common prodromal (warning) symptom, reported by nearly half to two-thirds of the patients. Musculoskeletal symptoms persist through the headache phase but often improve as the attack subsides. One woman knew her attack would end shortly after her neck symptoms resolved.

The neck pain typically affects the back of the neck on the same side as the headache in the region of the large occipitofrontalis muscle, which runs from the back of the head over to the forehead. Pain can also affect both sides of the neck, occasionally radiating into the shoulders.

Neck and back pain can also trigger attacks, particularly if they result from a specific injury. Even simple muscle tension from poor posture, sitting in front of a computer or driving a car, can be a cause. Physical causes such as these require physical treatments, although it may be several months before you see any benefit in reducing your migraine frequency.

Sometimes, over-enthusiastic osteopathy or physiotherapy can trigger attacks. Like exercise, a gentle start is the key to long-term benefit.

Temporomandibular joint dysfunction

If you find that your jaw 'clicks' when you eat or even locks out, or if you notice that you frequently wake with migraine after grinding your teeth at night, a visit to your dentist could resolve your migraine attacks. The dentist can adjust the bite with a device worn in the mouth at night.

Temporomandibular joint dysfunction, when you feel pain and tenderness in your jaw joints, can be associated with tension in the muscles controlling your jaw. This can give rise to a headache, often occurring daily, but occasionally triggering a migraine as well. One young girl with daily headaches and tender jaw joints found that all her symptoms resolved when she stopped chewing gum!

Travel

How often have you found that a long journey by car or aeroplane results in a migraine? Travel is associated with many potential migraine triggers: lack of sleep from the preparation for the trip and from the trip itself, stress, missed or delayed meals, and loud noises.

If you're travelling by plane, there are the added triggers of dehydration and cramped seats with little room to move. It remains uncertain as to whether pressure changes in aircraft trigger migraine, particularly with improved cabin pressures in most modern passenger aircraft.

Weather

For centuries, the seasonal hot dry winds around the world, such as the Swedish Föhn, the Mediterranean Meltemi and the Canadian Chinook, have been associated with headaches and general irritability. In other parts of the world, less obvious changes in barometric pressure have been cited as a trigger for migraine, although the data are conflicting.

In the UK, although a study in London found no evidence for an effect of weather on migraine, the results of a study in Scotland suggested that a rise in barometric pressure *was* associated with increased migraine frequency.

Weekends

Migraineurs who work from Monday to Friday often report that their migraine is more likely to occur at the weekend. This pattern is most likely to result from a gradual build-up of triggers during the week, culminating in an additional barrage of triggers at the weekend.

For example, you may feel more relaxed after a stressful week, go to bed late on Friday night after an evening out, sleep in on Saturday morning and change your eating patterns, often with a late breakfast. It is therefore not surprising that an attack of migraine results.

Caffeine withdrawal, following a reduced caffeine intake at weekends compared with the working week, has also been blamed. Many sedentary workers take unaccustomed exercise or physical activity at weekends, including housework, gardening and DIY projects.

Computers

Computers are often implicated as a cause of headache. The flickering screen usually gets the blame but, in fact, the more likely cause is related to how you sit and work at the computer. In addition to increased muscle tension in the head and neck, working at a computer for long periods results in a reduced blink rate and dry, sore eyes.

If you do get headaches or migraines after working at a computer for long periods of time, set an alarm to sound every half an hour to remind you to take a short break. Look at something as far into the distance as you can, blink your eyes hard several times, and try some simple and quick exercises to stretch your neck and shoulder muscles. Even just gently rolling your neck from side to back to side to front and stretching your arms out to the sides and above can make a great deal of difference.

Other causes

There are many other factors implicated in triggering migraine attacks. These include bright sunlight, strong smells, smoke-filled rooms, dehydration, going to the cinema and loud sounds.

KEY POINTS

■ Migraine triggers vary from person to person, and are not always the same for different attacks in the same person

■ Several triggers may work together to initiate an attack

■ Some triggers are more important than others

■ Important migraine triggers include insufficient food, hormonal fluctuations in women, too much or too little sleep, illness, and neck or back pain

Living with migraine: self-help

Lessening the impact

There is no known cure for migraine. However, you can do a great deal to lessen the impact of migraine by identifying and avoiding your specific triggers and by using effective treatments when necessary. Treatments can be symptomatic (to relieve the symptoms of a migraine attack) or prophylactic (to prevent a migraine attack occurring). By doing this you can move from a condition that is out of control to one that is under your control.

Both non-drug treatments and drugs can be used to treat and prevent migraine attacks. In most cases, preventive measures usually just reduce the frequency and severity of attacks rather than abolish them entirely.

Where to get information about migraine

In the UK, there are two charities that have been set up to help migraine sufferers: the Migraine Action Association and the Migraine Trust. More information about these groups is given at the end of the book under 'Useful information' (see page 161).

Internationally, the World Headache Alliance (WHA) is a global cooperative of more than 40 national lay organisations worldwide, including Migraine Action Association and Migraine Trust. In addition to its main aim of relieving people's suffering from headaches, WHA is also lobbying governments and raising awareness of headaches as a public health concern. Contact details are listed in 'Useful information' (page 161).

Disability from migraine

It goes without saying that, when you have an attack of migraine, you are pretty restricted in what you can do. This may not be such a problem if your attacks are infrequent but, when they start to occur regularly, your education, work, family and social activities can all suffer.

This can have severe implications such as loss of promotion or even unemployment, in addition to putting a strain on your relationships. Some people are very disabled by migraine because they are constantly in fear of the next attack – they find it hard to function normally, even when they don't have an attack.

Recognising these problems is not always easy. The MIDAS (see page 44) and HIT questionnaires are very useful tools that can help you, and other migraineurs, find out just how much migraine affects your life. You can download the MIDAS questionnaire from the internet or you can take the HIT test online (see 'Websites', page 169).

You can take the results to your doctor to help him or her understand the problem. In this way, you can work together to find an effective course of action for you.

The Migraine Disability Assessment Questionnaire (MIDAS)

Instructions

Please answer the following questions about ALL the headaches you have had over the last three months. Write your answer in the box next to each question. Write 0 if you did not do the activity in the last three months.

1. On how many days in the last three months did you miss work or school because of your headaches? .... ☐☐ days

2. On how many days in the last three months was your productivity at work or school reduced by half or more because of your headaches (do not include days you counted in question 1 where you missed work or school)? .... ☐☐ days

3. On how many days in the last three months did you not do household work because of your headaches? .... ☐☐ days

4. On how many days in the last three months was your productivity in household work reduced by half or more because of your headaches (do not include days you counted in question 3 where you did not do household work)? .... ☐☐ days

5. On how many days in the last three months did you miss family, social or leisure activities because of your headaches? .... ☐☐ days

MIDAS SCORE .... ☐☐

The Migraine Disability Assessment Questionnaire (MIDAS) (contd)

A. On how many days in the last three months did you have a headache? (If a headache lasted more than one day, count each day) .... ☐☐ days

B. On a scale of 0–10, on average how painful were these headaches? (Where 0 = no pain at all and 10 = pain as bad as it can be) .... ☐☐

© Innovative Medical Research 1997

The MIDAS Questionnaire has been developed to help you and others assess how migraine has affected you over the last few months. Complete Questions A and B first.

For Questions 1 and 2, work or school means paid work or, if you are a student, education at college or school.

For Questions 3 and 4, household activities include days lost by those in full-time home care or non-work/school days for those in paid employment. They should not include days counted in Questions 1 and 2.

For Question 5, consider additional days lost from all other activities.

Add up the numbers from Questions 1–5 and write them in the MIDAS score box. If your MIDAS score is greater than 10, it is recommended that you seek medical advice. However, irrespective of your MIDAS score, you should see your doctor if you have any concerns about your headaches. Questions A and B are not used to calculate the MIDAS score, but provide extra information that doctors may find useful in making their treament decisions.

What can you do to help yourself?

There is a great deal that you can do to treat migraine without needing to see a doctor, provided that you are sure of the diagnosis. Your pharmacist can advise you on the best treatments to take and when you should seek medical advice. There are also some simple measures that can make drugs more effective and help to prevent attacks.

Take drugs early ...

Always carry with you at least one dose of your preferred medication, so that you can take it as soon as you feel an attack coming on. It is important to take your medication early, as it is more likely to be effective. Your stomach is less active during a migraine, and so is less able to absorb drugs that you take by mouth (orally).

The problem is knowing whether you've got a migraine that needs treating rather than a headache that will resolve of its own accord. Some people find that, if they shake their head or put their head between their knees when a headache starts, they can tell that it will be a migraine because their head will throb. This will not occur if it is 'just a headache'.

... but not too often

Drugs can be very effective at controlling the symptoms of migraine, provided that they are taken correctly and not overused. It is important not to take symptomatic treatment too often because, if you start taking it on most days, you could end up giving yourself a headache.

This is because your body starts to get accustomed to the treatment and seems less able to control pain effectively. Consequently, headaches will be there

Categories of medication

The sale and supply of medicines are controlled by the Medicines Act 1968 and appropriate European Community Directives, and the body charged with administering the code is the Medicines Control Agency (MCA).

Products that are judged to be 'medicines' are classified according to, among other things, the status of their active ingredient(s):

- General sales list (GSL): many simple medicines can be bought from the shelves of a supermarket or general shop
- Pharmacy only (P): some medicines can be bought only from a pharmacist in a licensed pharmacy
- Prescription-only medicines (POM): other medicines with powerful actions and possible serious side effects are available only on prescription from your doctor

when you wake up on most days and these headaches respond less well to treatment.

To avoid this happening, you should never take drugs to treat headache symptoms regularly on more than two or three days a week. It doesn't matter if you take a small amount or the full recommended dose on those days – the important thing is that there are at least four consecutive days on which you don't take drugs.

If you find that you need to take drugs more often than this, even if it is just one or two doses a day, you must seek your doctor's advice. Taking symptomatic drugs on most days makes it hard for any other medication to work – the headaches become unresponsive because 'medication overuse headache' develops (see 'Chronic daily headaches', page 124).

This is different from when your doctor prescribes specific preventive drugs to take every day. These prophylactic (preventive) medications work in quite a different way from symptomatic treatments by preventing the migraine process from developing in the first place.

What treatment to take

Drugs to treat the symptoms of migraine are called symptomatic or acute treatments. Symptomatic drugs include painkillers bought from a pharmacy or supermarket, as well as drugs specifically developed for migraine, such as 'triptans', which are available on prescription (see page 63).

The pharmacy

Most painkillers contain aspirin, paracetamol or ibuprofen. For migraine, soluble or effervescent products work faster and are more effective than ordinary tablets. Mouth-dispersible preparations of aspirin, which you suck or chew, have been shown to be effective in recent clinical trials, and are particularly convenient because they dissolve in your mouth without the need for water.

Sometimes these drugs are combined with stronger painkillers such as codeine (a mild opiate drug) to make them more powerful, or with antihistamines, which help to reduce nausea or relieve muscle tension. Some tablets are more specifically designed for migraine. The pharmacist can advise you about these and how to take them safely. There is little difference between them, so which one you choose is a matter of personal preference.

For maximum effect, you should take the tablets as early in the attack as possible, although you should never take more than the maximum dose indicated. If none of the tablets is effective or you need more than the recommended dose, you should see your doctor.

Domperidone (also known as Motilium) is a powerful anti-sickness drug that enhances gut motility (movement), improving drug absorption. A dose of 20 milligrams of domperidone taken with a painkiller can treat both the headache and the accompanying sickness. It is recommended for migraine only on prescription from your doctor. However, an over-the-counter formulation (Motilium 10) can be purchased from pharmacies for treating nausea and vomiting, and also to treat indigestion resulting from reduced gut motility.

Other anti-sickness drugs can be useful, but these do not have the effect of enhancing gut motility. Prochlorperazine (Stemetil) has been tested in clinical trials in migraine, and a formulation that dissolves in your mouth (called Buccastem M) can be purchased over the counter (OTC) from pharmacies.

What to do during an attack

Try to eat something if you can, preferably after taking your drug. Bland food, such as dry toast or a biscuit, can sometimes ease nausea. If you do vomit, it is much less painful if you have eaten something than retching on an empty stomach. Some people prefer to eat something sweet, whereas others prefer to have a fizzy drink, such as lemonade, or a cup of tea with sugar.

In an ideal world, you should give in to the attack and try to rest. Sleep is nature's way of aiding your recovery – struggling on through the migraine usually only prolongs the attack. Obviously, not everyone can pack up work and go to bed, but you should at least try to take things more slowly. Catch up on more routine tasks rather than something that requires concentration.

Try putting a covered hot-water bottle or an ice pack on the back of your neck or on the most painful point – but do not leave it on for too long. Some people have found that listening to a relaxation tape or pressing on acupuncture points can help. You could cover your eyes with an eye mask – you can buy one from a pharmacy.

Although many migraineurs prefer to lie in bed, a few find it more comfortable to sit propped up in a chair. You should do whatever seems natural to minimise the pain.

Keep an attack diary
Controlling migraine is all about looking for patterns of attacks, so you should keep a record of when you get attacks. You need to record, either in a notebook or on a special migraine diary, the following information:

- Date of the attack

- What time the attack began

- Symptoms including aura, if these were present

- What medication you took, what dose and what time you took it

- What time the attack ended

- What the warning signs were.

Warning signs (premonitory symptoms) precede the headache by several hours, sometimes even during the evening or day before (see 'Different types of migraine', page 7). These subtle changes in your mood or behaviour can be present before attacks of migraine with or without aura.

You may not notice these symptoms until your attention is drawn to them and they are often more obvious to your friends and relatives than to you. Clumsiness, yawning, and feeling tired and irritable are common premonitory symptoms. Other symptoms include a stiff neck, feeling thirsty, and sensitivity to light and sound.

Recognising these premonitory symptoms can be of enormous benefit because avoiding known trigger factors during this time may be all that is necessary to stop the attack developing further.

Keep a trigger diary

Trigger diaries can help you to unravel the mystery of why you get attacks. Triggers are discussed in more detail under 'Migraine triggers' (page 28).

By being aware of a potential build-up of triggers, you can take extra care to minimise them. A few people are aware of at least some of their triggers. Others are confused when a suspect trigger sometimes results in an attack but doesn't have the same effect every time. This is because triggers usually act in combination, building up to a threshold and triggering the attack, so they need to look for other triggers.

Rather than 'What triggers an attack?', a more useful question is 'How many triggers do you need to initiate an attack?'. Even your usual daily routine can include triggers that you are not aware of, because you remain below the threshold of an attack until a few extra triggers crop up. It is important to keep a record of potential triggers every day, as you are unlikely to remember them clearly when you have an attack.

To keep a trigger diary, buy a small notebook and make a record of a typical day's routine, including mealtimes, travel, and work and leisure activities. Every evening, record any differences to your usual routine. Also run through a list of typical migraine triggers and record any that happened that day. Note any unusual changes in your mood or behaviour because these may be premonitory (warning) symptoms. Some of these, particularly food and chocolate cravings, are often confused with triggers.

If you take any regular medication, including vitamin, mineral or other supplements or complementary remedies, make a note of these. Similarly, record when you have a period, and any premenstrual symptoms that occur or when you take the oral contraceptive pill or hormone replacement therapy (HRT).

Identify and treat triggers

You should continue to complete the trigger diary until you have had at least five attacks. Compare the information in each and see whether there was a build-up of triggers coinciding with the attacks. Looking back on the attacks, were there any warning signs?

Study the list of the triggers that you've identified and divide them into two groups – those that you can do something about (for example, missing meals, dehydration) and those that are out of your control (for example, your menstrual cycle, travelling). First try to deal with the triggers over which you have some control. Cut out suspect triggers one at a time – if you try to deal with them all at once you will not know which are most relevant to you. Try to compensate – if you are having a particularly stressful time, take care to eat regularly and find ways to unwind before you go to bed.

If your attacks regularly start in the late morning or late afternoon, look at your mealtimes. A mid-morning or mid-afternoon snack may be all that is necessary to prevent the attacks. Similarly, if you have an early evening meal and wake with an attack, try a snack before you go to bed.

If you suspect that specific foods trigger your attacks, cut them out of your diet one at a time for a few weeks before reintroducing them. You will need to do this with the same food more than once, as a check.

If you think a large number of foods are involved, speak to your doctor. This is because you may risk causing malnutrition by cutting too many foods out of your diet – elimination diets should be supervised professionally.

Example of a migraine attack diary

Month .... Year ....

Name .... Date of birth.....................

Day	Day of week	Time attack starts	Did you have an attack? Headache/Migraine	Severity Mild/Moderate/ Severe	Feel sick Yes/No	Vomit Yes/No
1						
2						
3						
4						
5						
6						
7						
8						
9						
10						
11						
12						
13						
14						
15						
16						
17						
18						
19						
20						
21						
22						
23						
24						
25						
26						
27						
28						
29						
30						
31						

Please keep any other relevant notes on a separate sheet.

Other drugs: daily preventive: Name .... Dose................

Hormonal treatments: Name ....

Medication taken (please use additional paper if necessary)			Hormones taken Yes/No	Menstrual period Yes/No
Medication name	Time taken	DOSE		

Trigger diary example

The following may help in formulating a diary of
trigger factors:

Monday
No changes to usual routine

Tuesday
Skipped exercise class – too busy at work

Wednesday
Drove 65 miles to visit a client. Very hot journey.
Arrived back late so dinner was 2 hours later than
usual

Thursday
Woke up late so skipped breakfast
Busy day at work – missed exercise class again
Early night

Friday
Work OK, usual routine
Went to cinema in the evening
Late evening meal
Late to bed

Saturday
Slept in extra hour and a half
Skipped breakfast
Shopping

KEY POINTS

■ Both non-drug and drug treatments can be used to treat and prevent migraine

■ There are many self-help measures to treat migraine that do not involve seeing a doctor

■ Drugs that treat migraine attacks are called acute, or symptomatic, treatments, and include painkillers and drugs that stop nausea

■ Drugs used to prevent attacks (prophylactics) are available only on prescription and are discussed in the next chapter

■ Migraineurs should identify their triggers and make changes where they can (such as not missing meals)

■ They should also keep a diary of their attacks (see pages 50–6)

Living with migraine: seeing a doctor

When to see your GP

If you feel that you can manage your migraines yourself, there is obviously no need to see your doctor. But if you find that the treatments available from a pharmacy are not sufficiently effective, or if there is any doubt about the cause or nature of your headaches or if the pattern of your headaches changes, it is important to visit your doctor to make sure of the diagnosis.

Very few headaches are caused by anything serious, but they can sometimes be a symptom of an underlying medical problem. Do not think that you are wasting your doctor's time. It is much better to be reassured than worry that there is something wrong.

What information to take to your GP

Take your trigger and attack diaries with you, and a completed MIDAS questionnaire (see page 44). List the various treatments that you have already tried, how you took them and what effect they had.

Make a note of when your headaches first started and how they have changed over the years. This information will help your doctor to assess the problem more quickly and make it easier to tailor treatments to your individual needs.

As there are no tests for migraine, your doctor cannot tell whether the treatment that he or she suggests first is going to be the most effective, so be prepared for several visits. There is no cure for migraine, but an effective treatment can help you to regain control over the attacks.

Seeing a specialist

If your attacks do not follow the usual pattern of migraine or other primary headaches, it is likely that your doctor will refer you to a medical specialist such as a neurologist (nervous system specialist). Some clinics, such as the City of London Migraine Clinic (see page 161), have been set up to help migraine sufferers understand their condition and find ways of treating the causes, not just the symptoms. You don't need to have severe or frequent attacks to benefit from referral.

What your GP might prescribe

Your GP can advise on specific drugs that can be prescribed for migraine. Even if you have seen your doctor in the past with little success, it is worth going again because you may need to try more than one type of treatment before you find the one that suits you best. Also, new treatments are being developed all the time.

Your doctor can prescribe two types of drugs:

(1) those to treat an attack (acute or symptomatic treatment)

(2) those to prevent it (preventive or prophylactic treatment).

Don't be surprised if your doctor suggests drugs that you can buy from a pharmacy. It may be that you haven't been taking them at the right time or in the right dose, and making simple changes can make the same drugs more effective.

Drugs to treat an attack – acute treatment

There are many different treatments available, and your doctor can advise on which are likely to help you the most. You may find that you benefit from having a choice of several different medicines to take, depending on the severity of the attack at the time you treat it. For example, if you wake in the middle of a severe attack, you are best taking a specific migraine drug such as a triptan (see below if your GP has prescribed this type of drug).

If, however, you feel an attack coming on during the day, simple painkillers may be enough in the first instance, although, if they haven't worked within an hour, more specific treatments are usually necessary without further delay. Your doctor can advise on the safety of different drug combinations.

Prescription drugs

If simple painkillers are not effective, your GP may prescribe an anti-sickness drug, such as domperidone or metoclopramide, to help your usual painkillers to be absorbed into your bloodstream more effectively. These are available on prescription combined with either paracetamol or aspirin in a single tablet for convenience (MigraMax, Paramax).

Several prescription-only painkillers are prescribed for migraine, especially when a person's neck and shoulder muscles are tender during attacks. These are called non-steroidal anti-inflammatory drugs (NSAIDs) and include diclofenac, naproxen and tolfenamic acid. Some of these drugs are available as suppositories, which are particularly useful if vomiting makes you unable to take tablets.

There are also some drugs specific to the treatment of migraine, and these do not act as painkillers. They are thought to reduce the pain of a migraine headache by narrowing the swollen blood vessels and reversing the chemical changes in the brain that occur in migraine.

One of these, ergotamine, has been used for over 70 years. The others belong to a new class of drugs, the triptans (see page 63), which have been available since the early 1990s. Both ergotamine and triptans can be very effective for migraine but are not usually necessary for every attack.

If you need ergotamine or triptans to control severe attacks, you should take them as early as possible in the attack, waiting only one hour after you have failed to respond to other drugs. Their use is not recommended if you are pregnant or breast-feeding (see page 101).

Ergotamine

Ergotamine (compound tablets such as Cafergot and Migril) is now usually prescribed when simple painkillers or triptans are not effective. It is available as tablets (some of which dissolve under your tongue)

Using suppositories

Some drugs are available as suppositories, which are particularly useful if vomiting makes you unable to take tablets. If you experience side effects from a medication, try halving the dose.

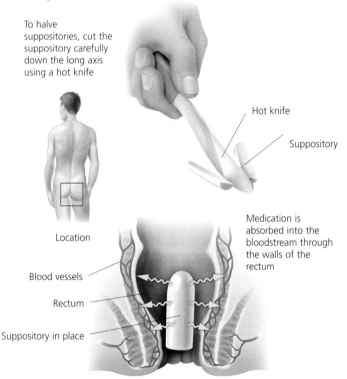

To halve suppositories, cut the suppository carefully down the long axis using a hot knife

Hot knife

Suppository

Location

Medication is absorbed into the bloodstream through the walls of the rectum

Blood vessels

Rectum

Suppository in place

and suppositories. Ergotamine can aggravate nausea and vomiting, particularly if the dose is too high.

This can be counteracted by taking an anti-sickness drug at the same time as you take the ergotamine. Dizziness and muscle cramps are other typical side effects. If you experience any of these symptoms, try taking a smaller dose, for example, half a tablet or half a suppository. To halve suppositories, cut the suppository in half down the long axis using a hot knife.

To gain maximum benefit from ergotamine, take it as soon as the migraine headache starts and use suppositories because the drug is best absorbed when given by this method. You should not exceed the recommended dose, because of the risk of ergotism (a condition causing gangrene of the fingers and toes, diarrhoea and vomiting) or ergotamine-induced headaches. Ergotamine should not be taken if you have uncontrolled high blood pressure or ischaemic heart disease, such as angina or a heart attack, because it can aggravate these conditions or if you are taking beta-blocker drugs.

Dihydroergotamine is reported to be as effective as ergotamine with a low incidence of the recurrence of migraine symptoms (so that attacks are shorter). Its main advantage over ergotamine is that it has similar but fewer unwanted effects.

Although it has been used for many years in several countries worldwide, it is currently not available in the UK since a nasal spray preparation (Migranal) was withdrawn. As with ergotamine, you should not use it if you have ischaemic heart disease or high blood pressure or are taking beta-blocker drugs for your migraine or high blood pressure, angina or anxiety.

Triptans

There are seven triptans, with six currently available: almotriptan (Almogran), eletriptan (Relpax), frovatriptan (Migard), naratriptan (Naramig), rizatriptan (Maxalt), sumatriptan (Imigran) and zolmitriptan (Zomig). These drugs act on specific parts of your brain that respond to serotonin. One way in which they are thought to treat migraine is by constricting only those blood vessels that become swollen during an attack, unlike ergotamine, which constricts blood vessels all over your body.

Although studies suggest that triptans are effective when taken at any stage of a migraine headache, they are probably most effective if you take them as soon as the headache starts. There appears to be little benefit from taking a triptan at the start of an aura – it is best to wait and take the triptan when the headache develops.

Possible side effects

Typical side effects include nausea, dizziness, fatigue and feelings of heaviness in any part of the body. These symptoms are usually short lasting.

Tightness and heaviness can also occur in your chest, which may make you worried about the effect of triptans on your heart. These 'chest' symptoms have been the subject of intense research to identify their cause and, in most cases, there is no evidence to suggest that they arise from the heart in healthy people.

'Chest' symptoms are of concern, however, if:

- you feel pain, rather than pressure, affecting your chest or arm

- they last longer than 60 minutes

- they begin to appear in later attacks, and you had no symptoms when you used the drug on the first few occasions.

Recurrence of the headache is a more difficult problem – the migraine attack is effectively treated, but the symptoms return later in the same day or the following morning. This can usually be resolved by taking a second dose of a triptan, although the attack can occasionally occur repeatedly over several days, particularly with menstrual attacks of migraine. Obviously it may not be appropriate to keep taking repeated doses of triptans for several days and, in these instances, other acute treatments may be better.

Who shouldn't take them?

Although triptans are safe and very effective in otherwise healthy migraineurs, certain people should not take them. These include people with ischaemic heart disease or uncontrolled hypertension (high blood pressure). If you are at a potential risk of heart problems (for example, a close family relative had a stroke or heart attack at an early age), or if you smoke or have diabetes, you should be checked carefully by your doctor before taking a triptan. Always make sure that your doctor knows what medicines you are currently taking before starting new medicines.

The different types of triptan
Sumatriptan

Sumatriptan (Imigran) was the first triptan to be developed and is available as a tablet (including a new rapidly dispersing tablet), a self-administered injection and a nasal spray. You should use a second dose only if the migraine has responded to the first dose, but your symptoms have returned. Sumatriptan should not be taken at the same time as ergotamine or other triptans or with certain antidepressant drugs known as monoamine oxidase inhibitors. It should be avoided if you are sensitive to sulphonamide antibiotics or are taking methysergide.

Almotriptan

Almotriptan (Almogran) is available as a tablet. It is a good all-rounder and is as effective at treating migraine headache as sumatriptan but with studies reporting no more side effects in people taking almotriptan than in those taking dummy treatments (placebo). Almotriptan should not be taken at the same time as ergotamine or other triptans. It also interacts with lithium, a drug sometimes used for cluster headache and more usually for bipolar disorder (manic depression). The drug should be avoided if you are sensitive to sulphonamide antibiotics or are taking methysergide.

Eletriptan

Eletriptan (Relpax) is available as a tablet. Clinical trials suggest that it may work more quickly than sumatriptan and may be more effective although with a similar likelihood of side effects. Eletriptan should not be taken at the same time as ergotamine, dihydro-ergotamine or by someone taking a course of certain antibiotics (erythromycin, clarithromycin), antifungals (ketoconazole and itraconazole) or anti-HIV drugs (ritonavir, indinavir and nelfinavir).

Frovatriptan

Frovatriptan (Migard) is available as a tablet. It may be associated with less relapse of migraine than many of the other triptans and has few reports of significant side effects, although it is slower to take effect. Frovatriptan should not be taken at the same time as ergotamine, methysergide or other triptans. It is generally not recommended for people also taking monoamine oxidase inhibitors.

Treatment to relieve the symptoms of migraine can be administered in several ways

There are many different types of acute (symptomatic) treatment available. Each has its own method of being taken. You may find that one way suits you better than the others.

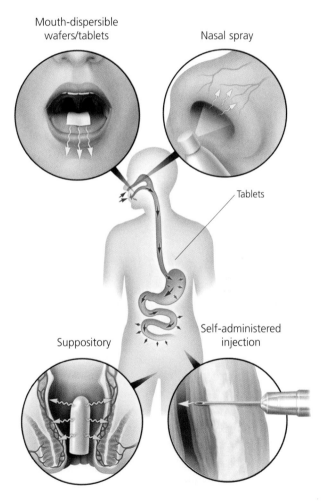

Mouth-dispersible wafers/tablets

Nasal spray

Tablets

Suppository

Self-administered injection

Naratriptan

Naratriptan (Naramig) is available as a tablet. It is slower to act than sumatriptan but has less marked side effects. It should also be avoided if you are sensitive to sulphonamide antibiotics or taking methysergide. Naratriptan should not be taken at the same time as ergotamine or other triptans.

Rizatriptan

Rizatriptan (Maxalt) is available as a tablet and as a mouth-dispersible, peppermint-flavoured wafer. The wafers are useful when water is not available. You should use a second dose only if your migraine symptoms return after the initial response. If you are taking the beta blocker propranolol, your doctor will prescribe a lower dose of rizatriptan. Rizatriptan should not be taken at the same time as ergotamine, methysergide or other triptans, and should be avoided if you are taking monoamine oxidase inhibitors.

Zolmitriptan

Zolmitriptan (Zomig) is presently available as a standard tablet, an orange-flavoured, mouth-dispersible tablet and a nasal spray. The last two formulations are convenient because you don't need water to take them. Zolmitriptan has the advantage over other triptans in that a second dose can be taken when the first dose is ineffective. Zolmitriptan should not be taken at the same time as ergotamine or other triptans. If you are taking monoamine oxidase inhibitors for migraine prevention or depression, you should use a lower dose. The drug should be avoided if you have certain heart rhythm defects, such as the Wolff–Parkinson–White syndrome.

Drugs to prevent migraine attacks
Common preventive treatments

You may need to take preventive, or prophylactic, drugs every day if you have attacks that cannot be adequately controlled with symptomatic medication. The aim of prophylaxis (prevention) is to help break the cycle of frequent or disabling attacks. However, no prophylactic medicine is 100 per cent effective – most reduce the frequency of attacks and/or make them shorter and less severe, so you will still need to take acute medication for breakthrough attacks.

For how long should you take them?

Although a few people need to take prophylactic medication in the long term, most people need to take it for only a course of three to six months. Most doctors recommend that you start with a low dose to minimise potential side effects. However, low doses are not effective for everyone. Therefore prophylactic drugs should not be deemed ineffective until you have tried what your doctor judges is an adequate dose for an adequate length of time.

This is usually a minimum of two weeks at the highest dose that does not produce unacceptable side effects. Although it is usual to prescribe just one drug for prophylaxis, it may be necessary to take two – propranolol and amitriptyline are typical examples of prophylactic drugs that are sometimes combined to give a greater effect.

It is very important to make sure that you take the drugs correctly, every day. If you have been prescribed a drug to take three times a day and find that you keep forgetting to take it, ask your doctor if there is a similar drug that you can take just once or twice a day instead. Make sure that you take the drugs at much the same time each day to ensure that the levels of the drugs in your bloodstream remain constant.

It is amazing how many people say that the drug is ineffective when they don't take it properly! The wrong diagnosis is another possibility – failure to respond to any prophylactic treatment is a common problem in people with medication overuse headaches, which develop with the overuse of symptomatic medication.

When stopping prophylactic medication, it is worthwhile gradually reducing the dose over a couple of weeks. This can help to reduce your fear of a resurgence of attacks.

Different types of preventive treatment
Beta blockers
Beta blockers (for example, metoprolol, nadolol, propranolol and timolol) are useful if stress is a trigger factor or if you have high blood pressure, but they should not be used in combination with ergotamine. Side effects include a lower tolerance to exercise, weight gain, fatigue (tiredness), sleep disturbance and cold extremities (such as your hands or feet). Beta blockers should not be taken if you have diabetes or asthma.

Antidepressants
Antidepressants (for example, amitriptyline) are particularly helpful if your sleep is disturbed or if migraine attacks are present when you wake up in the morning. Usually you will be prescribed a low dose to be taken at night.

Side effects may include a dry mouth, blurred vision, constipation and sedation. These are most apparent in the first two weeks and wear off as the drug starts to take

Preventive drugs used in the treatment of migraine attacks

There are a number of different drugs that can be used to prevent migraine. They all have potential side effects, some mild and others more severe, which your doctor will discuss with you.

Drug	Starting dose	Maximum daily
Beta blocker, e.g. propranolol	10 mg twice daily	240 mg in three divided doses (long acting, once daily)
Amitriptyline* (antidepressant)	10 mg at night	150 mg at night
Sodium valproate* (antiepileptic)	200 mg twice daily	1,000 mg twice daily
Topiramate (antiepileptic)	25 mg at night	50 mg twice a day

*Not licensed for migraine in the UK, but your doctor may like to prescibe them. Lack of a licence means that the drug's primary use is for a different condition. All the drugs listed have been shown to be effective in controlled clinical trials.

effect. For these reasons, it is necessary to persevere with the treatment for at least three weeks before assessing any side effects/benefits. Antidepressants should not be taken if you have a heart problem, epilepsy or glaucoma (increased fluid pressure in your eye).

Pizotifen

Pizotifen is a drug specifically used for the prevention of migraine. Although often prescribed in general practice, there is very little information to confirm its effectiveness. It can increase your appetite, so you need to watch your diet to make sure that you don't gain any weight.

Sedation (feeling drowsy) is another common problem, usually counteracted by taking the drug at night. For these reasons, it is rarely recommended by specialists to prevent migraine in adults.

Antiepileptics

Antiepileptics have been studied in migraine. As a result of their success in treating both conditions, they are increasingly called 'neuromodulators' rather than 'antiepileptics'. Sodium valproate is one such drug which has been used to prevent epileptic fits for many years and has also been shown to be an effective migraine prophylactic.

Although most migraineurs tolerate the drug with few problems, it can occasionally cause some nausea, stomach upsets, hair loss, tremor (shaking) and bruising. It cannot be taken if you have liver problems, so liver function tests should be performed before you start the treatment.

Sodium valproate should not be taken if you are pregnant or not using adequate contraception because its use in pregnancy is associated with well-documented abnormalities in an unborn baby. Although not licensed for migraine in the UK, sodium valproate is widely used by specialists and is licensed for migraine in the USA.

Topiramate has recently been licensed for migraine prevention after extensive clinical trials. These trials confirm its efficacy for migraine. Low doses are used to begin with, and they are gradually increased over several weeks until the maximum effective dose is reached. Side effects, such as tingling in the fingers, tiredness, weight loss, nausea and loss of appetite, are usual but genarally resolve with continued treatment.

In doses usually used to prevent migraine, topiramate does not appear to interact with combined hormonal contraception, although some doctors may still recommend the use of additional contraception if you are using this method. There is an increased risk of kidney stones developing during treatment with topiramate, which can be reduced by drinking plenty of fluids.

Gabapentin is a more recent 'neuromodulator' used by specialists for migraine prophylaxis, although not licensed for migraine. Common side effects include dizziness and tiredness. Weight gain is a limiting side effect.

Other drugs used to prevent the occurrence of migraine attacks

Methysergide (Deseril) is probably the most effective migraine prophylactic available, but it tends to be used only for people with severe attacks that have failed to respond to other drugs. This is because its use can, very rarely, increase the risk of developing scar tissue at the back of the abdomen (retroperitoneal fibrosis), around the heart valves and in the lungs. This is unlikely to occur if methysergide is stopped for at least one month after each six months of use. If identified early, the scar tissue formation often reverses.

Side effects of methysergide include nausea, dyspepsia (indigestion), leg cramps, dizziness and sedation. It should not be used if you have peripheral vascular disease (affecting the blood supply to your limbs), severe high blood pressure, heart disease, or impaired liver or kidney function. You should avoid taking ergotamine or dihydroergotamine for symptomatic treatment while taking methysergide.

Calcium channel antagonists, such as verapamil, are popular in some countries. They are not licensed for use in migraine in the UK.

Clonidine (Dixarit) is an old drug used for the management of hypertension (high blood pressure) and has shown limited effectiveness in migraine prevention. It may be useful in the management of menopausal women with migraine and hot flushes who do not wish to take hormone replacement therapy. It should not be taken by women with a history of severe depression because it can aggravate this.

Cyproheptadine (Periactin) is an antihistamine with anti-serotonin properties occasionally used in migraine. Side effects include sedation, weight gain, a dry mouth and dizziness.

KEY POINTS

■ You should see a doctor if over-the-counter treatments are ineffective, your headaches have not been diagnosed by a doctor or the pattern of your headaches changes

■ Your doctor may refer you to a specialist, such as a neurologist (nervous system specialist)

■ There are many different prescription drugs available to take during an attack to combat migraine symptoms (acute or symptomatic therapy)

■ Preventive or prophylactic treatments reduce the frequency of migraine attacks and must be taken regularly every day, usually for a three- to six-month course

Living with migraine: complementary treatments

The complementary approach

Nearly 70 per cent of migraine sufferers have tried 'alternative' or complementary treatments. Many of these treatments help to reduce the effects of triggers, especially neck and back problems, and can effectively control migraine, with or without medication. However, most of the following treatments are not available on the NHS and the cost of the treatment can vary considerably.

Physiotherapy

Chartered physiotherapists normally work with the medical profession. Look for the letters SRP or MCSP after the person's name, because these physiotherapists have at least three or four years of training. Some physiotherapists are qualified in acupuncture, electrotherapy and manual therapy, in addition to giving lifestyle training and advice.

Non-drug treatments for migraine

- Physiotherapy
- Osteopathy and chiropractic
- Acupuncture
- Homoeopathy
- Yoga
- Massage and aromatherapy
- Counselling and psychotherapy
- Alexander technique
- Biofeedback and relaxation
- Herbal remedies and vitamin supplements

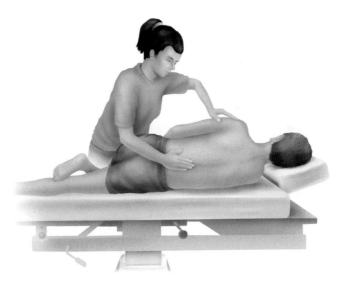

Physiotherapists, osteopaths and chiropractors can be useful
to treat back and neck problems and so help relieve
migraine in some people.

Osteopathy and chiropractic

Osteopaths and chiropractors treat problems relating to bones by manipulation. Registered osteopaths and chiropractors have completed a training course lasting several years and are skilled professionals.

They deal mostly with disorders of the spine and neck and their related muscles. Older people should be particularly careful with manipulation of their neck and spine, and should discuss this with their doctor before having a course of treatment.

Acupuncture

Acupuncture was developed thousands of years ago by Chinese physicians and involves the insertion of very thin needles into specific locations in the skin and underlying muscle. In all diseases, tender points develop on the surface of the body which disappear when the illness is cured. These are so-called acupuncture points.

Although these points can be spontaneously painful, most are usually only tender under pressure. Other recognised acupuncture points are not tender but are recognised by the experienced physician. The skin over these acupuncture points is pierced by a very fine needle, which is kept in place for a few minutes before it is withdrawn.

No one knows exactly how acupuncture works in preventing attacks of migraine but some sufferers find it very helpful. Pressing on tender points during an attack (acupressure) can also give relief.

You can find your acupressure points by gently pressing the muscles in your temples or down the back of your neck and shoulder. When you feel a tender point, painful on pressure, press gently. When starting

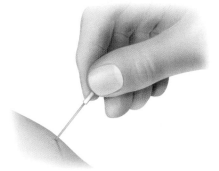

No one knows exactly how acupuncture works in preventing attacks of migraine, although some sufferers find it very helpful.

a course of acupuncture or acupressure, it is usually recommended to have one or two sessions a week for the first few weeks and then gradually reduce the frequency to maintain the effect.

Homoeopathy

The principle of homoeopathy is to treat 'like' with 'like'. Patients are prescribed minute doses of substances that can imitate the symptoms of their illness or medical condition. The substances recommended depend on the precise symptoms of the individual, so two people with similar problems may be given different treatments.

Homoeopathic treatments should be taken only on the advice of a qualified practitioner. There are several NHS homoeopathic hospitals in the UK, where patients are treated by medical doctors trained in homoeopathy, acupuncture and other complementary therapies.

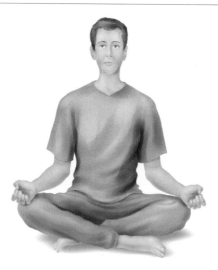

Some migraine sufferers find that regular yoga sessions relieve their symptoms.

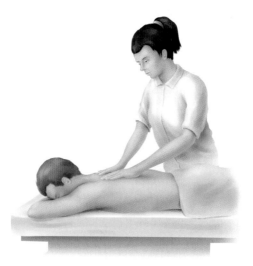

Massage can be very helpful in reducing tension in your muscles and achieving relaxation.

Yoga

Yoga stretches your muscles, relieves stress, helps your breathing and eases tension. It has been found to be helpful in relieving migraine by some sufferers. Many health clubs and fitness centres offer classes in yoga, and teach-yourself books and DVDs are readily available to buy.

Massage and aromatherapy

Massage can be very helpful in reducing tension in your muscles and achieving relaxation. If performed regularly, it can help to minimise headaches resulting from stress.

Some people find that massage combined with aromatic essential oils (aromatherapy) is particularly beneficial because essential oils can ease specific problems, including poor sleep or sinus pain. Studies using peppermint and eucalyptus oils have shown beneficial effects.

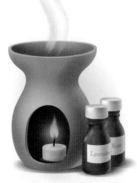

Aromatherapy combines massage with aromatic essential oils, which can ease specific problems.

Counselling and psychotherapy

Everyone has problems in life but not everyone is able to deal with them. Counselling or psychotherapy can help you to identify any stresses and find ways of dealing with them. As stress and anxiety can trigger migraine attacks, some people may find this type of treatment particularly beneficial.

Alexander technique

This technique was developed by F.M. Alexander in the 1920s. He believed that bad posture could trigger pain and illness.

The emphasis is on unlearning bad habits of movement and on correcting the relationship between your head and neck and the rest of your body. This treatment may be of specific help to headache sufferers with stiff and tender neck muscles.

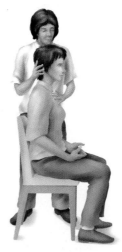

A practitioner of Alexander technique will show you how to correct the relationship between your head and neck and the rest of your body.

Biofeedback and relaxation

Biofeedback is a form of relaxation that teaches you to recognise the early signs of a migraine and how your body responds to them, so that you can stop the attack in its very early stages. To use biofeedback, you need to be trained to monitor changes in certain body functions, such as your heart rate, body temperature or muscle tension.

Once the training is complete, you are able to recognise your body's signals. By then reaching a state of relaxation, you can stop the muscle tension that triggers the attacks.

Herbal remedies and vitamin supplements

If you wish to take, or are already taking, a herbal preparation for confirmed migraine, or for any other diagnosed condition, you should seek the advice of a qualified practitioner who is a member of the National Institute of Medical Herbalists (NIMH). The NIMH is a regulating body for western herbal practitioners. Although herbal preparations can be extremely effective, it is important to remember that herbal is not the same as 'harmless' – many plants are highly toxic.

Hopefully, new legislation will enable herbal products to carry appropriate information on the packaging, so that they can be used safely without unnecessary concerns. Even when this information is made available, it is always best to err on the side of caution.

Feverfew

Studies show that the herb feverfew can prevent attacks of migraine. The herb is also known as *Tanecetum parthenium* and belongs to the daisy family. It is equally effective when taken as fresh leaves or

---

Avoid medicine interactions

Tell your doctor or pharmacist before you take any herbal preparation to ensure that the preparation is suitable for you, so that there are no unwanted effects.

If you are taking a herbal preparation, tell your doctor or pharmacist before you take any drugs that they recommend, to ensure that there are no unwanted interactions.

---

tablets. A daily dose of up to four leaves or 200 to 250 milligrams is usually sufficient, but any noticeable benefit may not be apparent for the first six weeks.

You may experience side effects, including mouth ulcers and stomach pain, or occasionally swollen lips. Pregnant or breast-feeding women should not take feverfew. As it has similar effects to aspirin (thinning the blood), it should not be used if you are taking other drugs regularly for this purpose, such as daily aspirin or warfarin.

Gingko biloba

This is a traditional Chinese medicine and has been used for menopausal symptoms, memory loss, depression and headaches. The effective dose is between 120 and 240 milligrams daily.

Reported side effects include dizziness, nausea, vomiting and headaches, which usually resolve with lower doses. *Gingko biloba* should not be used if you are pregnant or are planning a pregnancy. It also interacts unfavourably with warfarin, which is prescribed to thin the blood and prevent blood clotting.

St John's wort

St John's wort is a herb known to affect levels of the chemical serotonin in the brain. This chemical is involved in many conditions, including depression, anxiety and migraine.

Several recent controlled clinical trials have confirmed that St John's wort is as effective as conventional drugs in the treatment of mild-to-moderate depression, with the added benefit of fewer side effects. The doses used ranged from 300 to 1,050 milligrams daily, with the most recent study using 350 milligrams three times daily. These findings have resulted in St John's wort becoming a popular treatment for depression. In Germany, in particular, St John's wort outsells conventional antidepressants.

Historically, the preparation has also been used for the treatment of various types of mental illness and neuralgias (nerve pain). It is also known for its wound-healing properties. Many people with migraine have said that their migraine improves when they take St John's wort.

Studies have proved that the drug has few side effects in most healthy people. There have been a few reports of increased sensitivity to sunlight, but this effect is uncommon and is usually associated with the use of higher than recommended doses. There is also some information to suggest that St John's wort can stimulate the uterus (womb), so it is not recommended in pregnancy.

As a warning, St John's wort can interact with drugs used to treat migraine. The Committee on Safety of Medicines has issued a statement advising people taking triptans or a particular type of antidepressant called selective serotonin reuptake inhibitors or SSRIs (for example, Prozac), sometimes used in migraine, to stop taking St John's wort. This is because the combination may increase the level of serotonin in the body, increasing the likelihood of side effects, although the data are very limited.

The Committee on Safety of Medicines recommend that you stop St John's wort and continue taking triptans, as prescribed, and mention this to your doctor at your next routine visit. If you wish to continue taking St John's wort, you should make an early appointment with your doctor to discuss your prescribed medication. You should not stop taking your prescribed medication without your doctor's advice.

Vitamin B$_2$ (riboflavin)

High doses of riboflavin (vitamin B$_2$) of 400 milligrams daily (at least 250 times the recommended daily intake) have been shown to be effective for migraine prevention in controlled clinical trials. In these trials, the side effects were minimal with only one patient taking riboflavin leaving the study, because of drug-related diarrhoea. However, the long-term safety of taking such high doses of riboflavin has not been established and you should not take these doses without your doctor's advice.

Magnesium

Several studies have observed that people with migraine have low magnesium levels in their body, particularly women with premenstrual symptoms, and that increasing the body's magnesium levels with supplements may help migraine symptoms.

One study used 600 milligrams of magnesium dicitrate daily with good effect and minimal side effects. Magnesium sulphate, magnesium hydroxide and magnesium oxide preparations should be avoided because of their laxative effect.

Butterbur/Petasites

Petasites hybridus (butterbur) is a shrub found throughout Europe. The active component is thought to be petasin, a sesquiterpene ester with anti-inflammatory, anti-allergy and muscle-relaxing properties.

Several studies comparing daily butterbur against dummy capsules (placebo) have shown a reduction in migraine frequency in up to 45 per cent of sufferers compared with only 15 per cent of those taking placebo. The butterbur plant contains pyrrolizidine alkaloids, which have been associated with liver toxicity, although most supplements in the UK have removed the alkaloids.

However, concerns remain about the certainty that they have all been removed. The dangers of exposure to low levels of these alkaloids is unknown. The recommended dose is 25 mg twice daily.

Coenzyme Q10

A coenzyme is a substance needed for the proper functioning of an enzyme, which speeds up the rate at which chemical reactions take place in the body. Coenzyme Q10 is a compound that is made naturally in the body and studies comparing placebo coenzyme Q10 have shown a significant reduction in migraine frequency.

There are no serious reported side effects, although some people experience mild insomnia, raised levels of liver enzymes, rashes, nausea and upper abdominal pain. Other reported side effects have included dizziness, visual sensitivity to light, irritability, headache, heartburn and fatigue.

Certain drugs, such as those that are used to lower cholesterol or blood sugar levels, may reduce the effects of coenzyme Q10. Coenzyme Q10 may also alter the body's response to warfarin and insulin. Recommended doses vary between 150 mg and 300 mg daily.

Other remedies

Ginger and peppermint in any form can help to reduce the feelings of nausea associated with migraine and can help digestion. Lavender oil rubbed on to your temples is another soothing remedy.

KEY POINTS

■ Many migraineurs try complementary (alternative) therapies to ease their symptoms

■ Popular therapies include osteopathy and chiropractic, acupuncture, homoeopathy, yoga, massage and aromatherapy, and the Alexander technique

■ Feverfew is a herbal remedy often taken for migraine; another useful herb is St John's wort

Headaches in women

Are headaches more common in women?

It is an unfortunate fact of life that most headaches are more common in women than in men, although this difference between the sexes is most apparent during the reproductive years. The obvious reason for this is that female sex hormones play an important role, although they are not the only factor, and women should also read the next chapter on headaches in adults of both sexes.

The effect of hormones on headaches

Few studies have looked at the effect of hormones on non-migraine headaches, but studies of women attending the City of London Migraine Clinic show that women are more prone to non-migraine headaches around the time of their period, even if they also suffer from migraine. Headaches are also a recognised symptom of premenstrual syndrome (PMS, see page 96) and the menopause (page 103).

Some women notice that they experience more headaches when they start taking the oral contraceptive pill. These headaches usually settle after a few months, but occasionally it is necessary to change to a different type of pill. Apart from these specific events, hormonal changes have little effect on non-migraine headaches.

Migraine and hormonal changes

Research in Sweden showed that both sexes were equally prone to migraine until the age of 11, after which time girls were affected more than boys. Once a woman has had her first migraine, she is more likely to continue having attacks throughout the rest of her reproductive years. By the time the children in the original Swedish study had reached the age of 30, 70 per cent of the affected women continued to have migraine attacks compared with only 48 per cent of the men. The attacks usually become less frequent in both sexes after the age of 55.

Menstrual migraine

In a study at the City of London Migraine Clinic, 50 per cent of women felt that their migraine attacks were linked to their menstrual cycle. Fifteen per cent of the women questioned reported that they had experienced their first attack of migraine in the same year as their first menstrual period.

These initial attacks are often irregular, occurring at any time of the menstrual cycle, but by the time a woman reaches her mid to late 30s, she may notice that the attacks follow a monthly pattern. Sometimes this pattern becomes apparent only when her periods return after the birth of a baby.

In the same study we found that fewer than 10 per cent of women regularly had attacks of migraine within the two days before their period started and within the first few days of bleeding (days −2 to +2 of their cycle) and at no other time of the month. This coincides with the phase of the menstrual cycle when the concentrations of the hormones oestrogen and progesterone fall to their lowest levels. As a result of this research, we defined a migraine occurring on or between the two days before a period starts and the first few days of bleeding as 'menstrual migraine'.

A larger group of women, 35 per cent, regularly had attacks linked to menstruation but also had other attacks that occurred at any time of the month. We called this 'menstrually related migraine'. The

Migraine and the menstrual cycle

Research shows that migraine headaches occur most frequently in the day or two preceding the start of menstruation or during the first few days of a period.

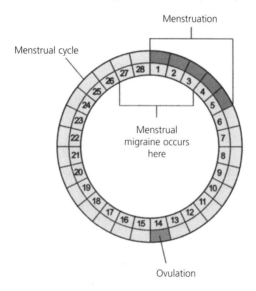

distinction between these two groups is important because, although hormonal factors play a role, women with 'menstrually related migraine' are also susceptible to non-hormonal triggers.

Menstrual migraine has been linked to the fluctuations in oestrogen levels that occur naturally during the menstrual cycle. There is no need to do any tests to check the hormones in these women because there is nothing wrong – they just seem to be more sensitive to normal hormonal fluctuations.

Hormones are not the only factors responsible, however. Although oestrogen supplements can prevent the drop in oestrogen, studies show that this treatment is not effective for every woman with menstrual migraine. The levels of other chemicals change throughout the menstrual cycle, such as prostaglandins, which are released just before and

Fluctuations in oestrogen levels

Menstrual migraine has been linked to the fluctuations in oestrogen levels that occur naturally during the menstrual cycle.

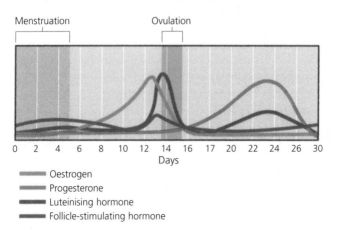

Oestrogen

Progesterone

Luteinising hormone

Follicle-stimulating hormone

during the menstrual flow. These other chemicals may be an important trigger, particularly for women who experience migraine on only the first or second day of bleeding.

Other non-hormonal triggers can also be important in menstrual migraine. Studies show that the changing levels of hormones affect sensitivity to other migraine triggers – for example, women are more susceptible to the effects of alcohol and missing meals around the time of their period.

Self-help

If you suspect a link between your periods and your migraine attacks, the first thing to do is to keep a diary (see pages 50–6). This helps to establish the exact relationship of the timing of the attacks and the different stages of your menstrual cycle.

Keep a note of any premenstrual symptoms, such as a craving for sweet foods, breast tenderness, etc., as well as an accurate record of the migraine attacks and your periods. For each attack, jot down the time it started, how long it lasted and what symptoms you experienced. Also keep a note of what treatment you took, what time you took it and how effective it was. Mention if the period was unusually painful or heavy. Also keep a note of any non-hormonal triggers that could have been responsible, as listed in 'Migraine triggers' (page 28).

After a few months, look back over your records and see if you can detect any patterns. Look especially at the non-hormonal migraine triggers, because avoiding these premenstrually may be sufficient to prevent what appears to be a hormonally linked attack. For instance, you should take care not to get overtired and, if necessary, cut out alcohol. Eat small, frequent snacks to keep your blood sugar level up because missing meals or going too long without food can trigger attacks.

Unfortunately, few effective treatments have been identified specifically for menstrual migraine, although vitamin B_6 is often suggested (it is an effective treatment for PMS – see below). It is advisable to seek the advice of a pharmacist or doctor before taking vitamin B_6 in high doses, because of the risk of possible toxic side effects in some people (for example, nerve damage).

Other over-the-counter treatments include evening primrose oil, which is effective for premenstrual breast tenderness in doses of up to 1.5 grams twice daily, and magnesium supplements, useful for other premenstrual symptoms including headache and migraine.

What can your GP do to help?

You should see your doctor for advice if you have severe symptoms or if the attacks remain unchanged after trying self-treatment for a few months.

Many women with hormonal migraine wonder why doctors do not perform any tests. The simple answer is that no tests are currently available that can direct a doctor to the cause of the problem, because all the standard hormone tests are usually normal. Studies measuring hormone levels have failed to identify any differences between women with migraine triggered by hormonal changes and women without migraine.

This is the same situation with all migraine triggers – there appears to be an increased sensitivity to normal events such as natural fluctuations in female hormones, missed meals and bright sunlight. This means that treatment, to a certain extent, becomes a matter of trial and error. However, depending on the stage of your cycle at which the attacks are occurring, some specific treatments are more likely to be effective than others.

Migraine may be associated with the premenstrual syndrome (PMS), a common condition in which women develop tiredness, irritability, breast tenderness and gain in weight from fluid retention in the few days before menstruation. This premenstrual migraine may respond to non-hormonal treatments available on prescription such as fluoxetine (Prozac). Hormonal treatments, such as the combined oral contraceptive pill or the injectable contraceptive Depo-Provera, can work by 'switching off' the normal menstrual cycle, because premenstrual migraine may be the result of the natural fall in oestrogen that occurs at this time of your cycle.

Alternatively, the attacks may be prevented with extra oestrogen, such as 1.5 milligrams of oestradiol gel daily or 100-microgram oestradiol patches changed every three and a half days, used from three days before the start of your period for a total of about seven days. This treatment has no effect on fertility because it supplements oestrogen levels only at a time when they are naturally falling and there is no evidence that it would have an adverse effect on pregnancy, although it is not recommended for use by women if they are trying to conceive.

Using oestrogen supplements in this way is different from hormone replacement therapy (HRT – see page 104) in which oestrogen is replaced throughout the cycle. Furthermore, additional hormones such as progestogen, used in HRT to protect the lining of the womb from overthickening in response to oestrogen,

Supplementing oestrogen using a skin patch

Premenstrual migraine that is caused by the natural fall in oestrogen may be prevented with extra oestrogen. The extra oestrogen can simply be absorbed into the body from skin patches.

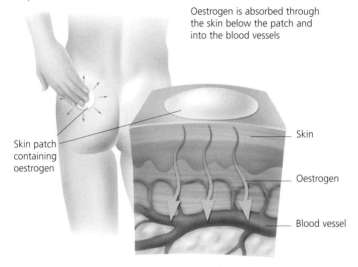

Oestrogen is absorbed through the skin below the patch and into the blood vessels

Skin patch containing oestrogen

Skin

Oestrogen

Blood vessel

are unnecessary because women continuing to have regular periods are producing their own protective natural progestogen, progesterone.

For migraine that occurs only during your period, particularly if your periods are also painful or heavy, it may be worth trying a drug that inhibits the release of prostaglandins. The most commonly used drug with this effect is mefenamic acid, which is available on prescription. This drug should be taken three to four times daily from the start of your period, for up to seven days. The advantage of this is that women with irregular periods can use it.

The Mirena intrauterine system is a contraceptive device inserted into your uterus (womb) where it releases small amounts of progestogen locally, stopping the lining of your uterus from thickening in response to oestrogen. This means that, in addition to its contraceptive action, using the Mirena system results in lighter and less painful periods. It has been interesting to note that several women using Mirena also report an improvement in their migraine that had previously been associated with menstruation.

What if it doesn't work?

If your attacks continue after trying a treatment for three cycles, do not give up hope. As your doctor cannot do any tests to identify the cause of hormonally related migraine, it is necessary to try different medications to treat different possible mechanisms. So if one treatment does not work, go back to your doctor and try another.

There are many other treatments that affect your hormonal cycle, including drugs that provoke a medical menopause, switching off the hormonal cycle in your brain. Unfortunately, side effects restrict the use of these drugs and they are usually prescribed only by gynaecologists (specialists in women's health).

Contraception
Combined oral contraceptives

Headaches are a common side effect of standard combined oral contraceptives, but they often improve with the continued use of the pill. They are related to the dose and type of hormones, and studies show that a headache is reported less often in users of the lowest dose pills (20 micrograms of oestrogen) containing newer 'third-generation' progestogens. Headaches mostly occur during the first few cycles of use, gradually resolving by the sixth cycle onwards.

Women who have migraine attacks before they start the pill often notice that they get their migraine during the pill-free interval, the time when their hormone levels drop to produce a withdrawal bleed. Changing to a different type of pill can sometimes help.

Taking a natural oestrogen supplement in the pill-free interval can also help, but the withdrawal bleed will still occur. Otherwise, taking two or three packets of the pill continuously before a pill-free interval can reduce the frequency of attacks.

A few women take the pill continuously and never take a break. Their migraines are often resolved but, because there is no controlled withdrawal bleed, unpredictable breakthrough bleeding can be a problem. There is little evidence that the monthly breaks from the pill are associated with any added health benefits over continued use of the pill, and the benefits of reduced menstrual problems and increased efficacy are clear. It is interesting to note that many female doctors take the pill continuously!

Migraine, the pill and the risk of stroke

The pill is very safe for most women who take it, including those who have migraine without aura, although not for those who have migraine with aura for the reasons discussed below. The pill also has many added benefits, such as reducing menstrual problems and premenstrual syndrome and reducing the overall risk of cancer.

Despite this well-established safety record, there are a few women for whom the risks of taking the pill outweigh the benefits. These are women who, for example, have high blood pressure or smoke heavily.

This is because they already run a higher risk of developing a stroke compared with healthy women, and this risk is further increased by taking the pill.

More recently, migraine with aura has also been associated with an increased risk of stroke in young women, although, in real terms, this risk is extremely small. However, studies show that this risk is more than five times greater when women with migraine with aura take the combined pill, compared with pill users who do not have migraine.

As a result of this risk, some authorities consider that the pill should not be given to women who have migraine with aura, particularly because there are now many alternative reversible methods of contraception, several of which, with the exception of the standard progestogen-only pill in women under age 35, are even more effective than the pill (see below). Similarly, if a woman with pre-existing migraine without aura develops aura after starting the pill, she should stop taking it immediately and seek medical advice – particularly as she may also need emergency contraception if she has had unprotected sex.

Other methods of contraception

Progestogen-only methods of contraception (such as the progestogen-only pill, Depo-Provera injections, implants and the Mirena intrauterine system) are not associated with an increased risk of stroke and are a safe alternative for women with any type of migraine. They can have varying effects on migraine, but the evidence suggests that, if the method results in 'switching off' ovulation and periods, the migraine usually improves.

Women using copper intrauterine devices may notice that they are more likely to experience migraine with their period, particularly if their periods become heavier. They may choose to switch to another method of contraception.

Pregnancy and breast-feeding

Studies suggest that between 60 and 70 per cent of female migraineurs experience an improvement in the frequency and severity of their attacks of migraine during the latter part of pregnancy, although both may be worse for the first few months. The reason for the improvement in established pregnancy is thought to be that the levels of oestrogen are more stable. However, it is unlikely that the true mechanism is so simple because there are many physical, biochemical and emotional changes in pregnancy that could account for improvement, including the increased production of the body's natural painkillers, muscle relaxation and altered blood sugar balance.

Women who have attacks of migraine without aura before becoming pregnant, particularly if they have noticed a link between migraine and their periods, are most likely to notice a respite from migraine during pregnancy. This typically continues during breast-feeding until their periods return, although migraine associated with the sudden drop in oestrogen immediately after giving birth is not uncommon. However, not every woman who has migraine without aura finds that her attacks improve during pregnancy – around 16 per cent continue to have attacks throughout.

In contrast to migraine without aura, women who have pre-existing migraine with aura are more likely to continue to have attacks during pregnancy. Also, if migraine starts for the first time during pregnancy, it is likely to be *with* aura.

There is no evidence that migraine, either with or without aura, has any effect on the outcome of a pregnancy or on the baby's growth and development. Many pregnant women favour non-drug methods of management while they are pregnant, particularly once they are aware that their migraine is likely to improve.

Early pregnancy symptoms can aggravate migraine attacks. Pregnancy sickness, particularly if it is severe, can reduce a woman's food and fluid intake resulting in low blood sugar and dehydration. Try to eat small, frequent carbohydrate snacks and drink plenty of fluids during pregnancy. Adequate rest is important to counteract over-tiredness. Other preventive measures that can be tried safely include acupuncture, biofeedback, yoga, massage and relaxation techniques (see page 77).

Few drugs have been tested for safety in pregnancy and during breast-feeding because of the obvious concerns. This lack of data means that manufacturers do not generally recommend the use of any drug in pregnancy, although this does not mean that they cannot be used. However, drugs should be considered only if the potential benefits outweigh the potential risks, which are difficult to assess because of the lack of data. Many drugs are most dangerous to the unborn child during the first three months, often before a woman knows that she is pregnant.

If you need to take migraine treatments during pregnancy, paracetamol is safe to take throughout pregnancy and breast-feeding. Aspirin is not recommended for pain relief during pregnancy, because it can cause problems with bleeding; therefore you should not take it without your midwife's or doctor's advice.

Non-steroidal anti-inflammatory drugs (NSAIDs) such as diclofenac, ibuprofen and naproxen are not recommended during the third trimester of pregnancy. Prochlorperazine has been used for pregnancy-related nausea for many years. Metoclopramide and domperidone have also been widely used during pregnancy in compound preparations to relieve nausea and pain by improving absorption of painkillers, but metoclopramide should not be used during breast-feeding. For severe attacks, your doctor will check that you are not dehydrated and could give you chlorpromazine for emergency treatment.

For continuing frequent attacks of migraine, which warrant daily preventive treatment, the beta blockers metoprolol and propranolol have the best evidence of safety.

The menopause

In the years leading up to a woman's final period (the menopause), her ovaries produce diminishing amounts of oestrogen. During this time of hormonal imbalance, it is not unusual for her migraine attacks to become more frequent or severe.

The few studies that have been undertaken suggest that the menopause aggravates migraine in up to 45 per cent of women, between 30 and 45 per cent do not notice any change and about 15 per cent notice an improvement. At least some of the increase in headaches around the menopause is not directly caused by hormones; women experiencing frequent night sweats may lose sleep, and over-tiredness is known to be a migraine trigger.

For most women, migraine settles after the menopause. This is possibly because the hormonal fluctuations cease – the oestrogen level is lower and more stable. However, a few women continue to have regular attacks after the menopause.

Hysterectomy

There is no evidence to suggest that a hysterectomy (removal of a woman's uterus and sometimes ovaries) is of any benefit in the treatment of hormonal headaches. The normal menstrual cycle is the result of an interaction between several different organs in a woman's body. These include organs in her brain, in addition to her ovaries and uterus.

Removing the uterus alone has little effect on the hormonal fluctuations of the menstrual cycle even though the periods cease. Removing the ovaries does affect oestrogen levels but there has been no study of the effect of oestrogen replacement therapy on migraine. It seems likely, however, that oestrogen replacement therapy might help to control symptoms in women with migraine who have had a hysterectomy.

Hormone replacement therapy

Hormone replacement therapy (HRT) replaces the oestrogen that the ovaries stop producing after the menopause. It is given to treat hot flushes, night sweats and other menopausal symptoms, including headaches, caused by the sudden loss of oestrogen. If HRT is taken for several years it has other benefits, such as reducing the risk of osteoporosis and bone fractures.

Women starting HRT later in life are at increased risk of heart disease, strokes and venous thrombosis. Most doctors recommend that you start HRT around the menopause and take it only for a few years. Taken in this way, the benefits of HRT outweigh potential risks.

KEY POINTS

■ Some women find that their headache or migraine worsens around the time of their period (menstrual migraine) or is associated with premenstrual syndrome (PMS)

■ There are no specific tests for menstrual migraine

■ Hormonal treatments, such as the combined oral contraceptive pill, may improve migraine in some women but in others migraine can worsen or aura can develop – in which case an alternative method of contraception should be considered

■ Many women discover that their migraine attacks become more frequent or severe in the years leading up to the menopause and then reduce in frequency and severity after the menopause

■ Hormone replacement therapy, if given in the right dose and by the right route (usually non-oral), can often help perimenopausal migraine

Headaches in adults of both sexes

A problem for both sexes

All epidemiological studies confirm that tension-type headaches and migraine are more common in women – studies in Denmark showed that tension-type headache affected 86 per cent of women and 63 per cent of men each year, with migraine reported by 16 per cent of women and 5 per cent of men each year. However, men also suffer from headaches and, just like many women, do not receive the attention and treatment that they need. Perhaps this is even more the case for men because the incorrect notion that headaches are 'all in the mind' carries a greater stigma for them.

Fortunately, this notion is changing, as it is recognised that many headaches result from specific changes in brain chemistry. Furthermore, specific treatments have been developed that have changed the lives of many migraine sufferers.

Puberty

Boys particularly seem to suffer from migraine during the growth spurt at puberty. Parents will notice that they seem to be forever buying larger sizes of clothes or shoes. At this time of life, a good diet with regular meals is often all that is necessary to prevent migraine attacks, as well as taking medicines to control the symptoms.

Exercise

Sport is also a common trigger in teenagers and even adults, particularly sustained physical exercise such as competitive sports. The migraines can often be prevented by drinking plenty of fluids to avoid dehydration and eating snacks or glucose sweets to maintain energy levels. Minor blows to the head during sport, such as heading a football or a hit on the face in a rugby tackle, can trigger an instantaneous migraine aura, not always followed by a headache. Although these attacks can usually be attributed to migraine, it is sensible to check with a doctor that there are no other underlying causes.

Work

Work and the working environment can trigger migraine attacks, as well as other headaches, particularly badly set up work-stations that create muscular strain, bad lighting, inadequate ventilation, etc. Work can suffer and migraine is a significant cause of reduced productivity and sick leave. Time pressures and other stresses at work may be significant triggers that are further affected by frequent migraine attacks. Some organisations employ occupational health specialists, who should be the first contact and who can often help to remedy many of the underlying causes. If your employer does not offer advice on occupational health, you should in the first place talk to your GP.

Other causes

Headaches – both migraine and other types – can also be a symptom of alcoholism, drug abuse, depression and marital conflicts in both sexes, and in these instances they will respond only to a resolution of the underlying cause.

Headaches more commen in men

A few types of headache affect men more than women, for example, headache associated with sex, which is also more common in those who have migraine or high blood pressure (see 'Other causes of headaches', page 140). Cluster headache is a rare type of headache that typically affects men (see 'Cluster headache and chronic paroxysmal hemicrania', page 131).

KEY POINTS

- Headaches and migraine are less common in men than in women

- Boys may experience headaches during their growth spurt at puberty

- Migraines associated with sport can often be prevented by drinking plenty of fluids and eating regular snacks for energy

- People may suffer from headaches if they are under stress at work or sit at a badly set up workstation

Headaches in children

Headaches are common in young people, affecting up to 60 per cent of children and teenagers. They are rarely a cause for concern, with obvious triggers such as missed meals, dehydration, tiredness or over-excitement, and readily respond to avoidance of the triggers or the treatment of the underlying cause.

Migraine in young people

Migraine is often missed in children, in whom it accounts for five to ten per cent of headaches, with an increasing prevalence in girls after puberty. It is important to recognise migraine in children for the following reasons:

- Migraine can be an important cause of time lost from school with obvious effects on education and long-term achievement.

- Migraine can be treated and prevented.

- Children who receive early education in migraine management continue to use these methods effectively as adults.

Is it migraine?

Recurrent bouts of headaches with nausea or vomiting, with complete freedom from symptoms between attacks, may be migraine. Some children also look pale and yawn a few hours before the headache starts; others are bursting with extra energy. A few children experience a visual aura before the headache, which they can often draw better than they can describe. Vomiting or sleep typically resolves the attack, often surprisingly quickly.

Although these symptoms are very similar to adult migraine, there are important differences:

- Attacks are shorter in children, sometimes lasting for less than an hour.

- The headache is typically all over the child's head rather than one sided.

- A headache may be only a minor symptom.

- Nausea, vomiting and abdominal pain are more prominent symptoms.

A diary can be useful to confirm the pattern of attacks and help children identify warning symptoms.

Abdominal migraine

Children have described abdominal migraine as 'a headache in my tummy' because the headache is often mild or absent. Unless the regularity of attacks is noticed, abdominal migraine is often misdiagnosed as gastroenteritis (a stomach upset), so the child misses out on effective treatment.

However, abdominal pain is a symptom of many other medical conditions affecting children, including irritable bowel syndrome or even coeliac disease (gluten intolerance). Therefore, any child with recurrent abdominal pain should be seen by a doctor to exclude other causes before labelling the symptoms as migraine.

Cyclical vomiting syndrome

Cyclical vomiting (recurrent attacks of vomiting lasting several days) is probably a variant of abdominal migraine. As a child can become extremely dehydrated with recurrent attacks of persistent vomiting, hospital admission is sometimes necessary to restore fluids. Fortunately, effective anti-sickness medication can often reduce the severity of attacks.

Probable causes

Just as in adults, migraine in children is triggered by a combination of factors, not just a single factor, and the same types of triggers apply (see 'Migraine triggers', page 28). Children are often aware of relevant triggers themselves: typically a lack of sleep, exercise, delayed or missed meals, and worries about home or school. Parental conflicts or bullying can be important triggers in children and can be easily overlooked. As in adults, diaries can be very useful in identifying how triggers accumulate over time. Children can also learn which situations are more likely to provoke attacks, enabling them to treat the attacks early on.

Inadequate nutrition is probably the major trigger in children, particularly during the teenage growth spurt. Parents should make an effort to provide their children with a proper breakfast and ensure that they have adequate meals and snacks during the school day. Constipation is often missed as a cause of headache and few parents are aware of their children's bowel habits. Constipation can usually be remedied by increasing a child's dietary fibre intake (for example, from fruit and vegetables) and fluid intake, although a gentle laxative may occasionally be necessary.

Food allergy or intolerance may be a trigger in a few children who have shown a definite and reproducible relationship between eating certain foods and the onset of migraine. In these cases, referral to a specialist may be valuable. However, for most children it is unnecessary to restrict food, even chocolate! Children often eat chocolate and are then too full to eat a proper meal. The real trigger is the missed meal – a change in routine rather than the chocolate.

Sport is a common trigger in children. Taking glucose tablets before and during sport can help, in addition to a half-time snack, with lots of fluid to

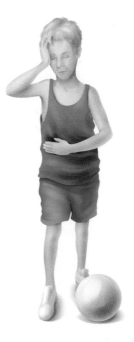

prevent dehydration. As in adults, minor blows to the head can also set off a migraine attack.

Travel triggers migraine as well as motion sickness, and this is often helped by eating small frequent snacks, sitting by an open window and making regular stops.

Treating the symptoms

The management of migraine is often inadequate in children, despite the fact that many children have to go to bed during an attack or experience attacks severe enough to make them cry with the pain.

Simple non-drug treatments, such as resting in a quiet, darkened room, using either a hot or cold pack – whichever the child prefers to ease the pain and gentle massage – may be enough to control mild symptoms. Most children want to lie down during an attack and they should be encouraged to sleep because this can hasten their recovery.

Drug treatment should be kept simple. If taken early in an attack, over-the-counter painkillers may be all that is necessary. It is important that the painkillers are specifically formulated for the child's age group. Junior syrups can be given to young children. Older children and teenagers may find that soluble or effervescent painkillers dissolved in a sweet fizzy drink are more palatable and more effective. The treatment should be taken in adequate doses as early in an attack as possible.

Junior paracetamol is often considered to be the drug of choice because it can be given as syrup to even very young children. It is also available as a suppository. Junior ibuprofen is a more effective alternative. Aspirin is not recommended for children aged under 16 in the UK because its use in children has been linked to a rare liver and brain disorder called Reye's syndrome. Migraleve is an over-the-counter tablet for children aged over 10, combining paracetamol, codeine and buclizine, which can help nausea. Children should avoid drugs containing caffeine.

If painkillers are inadequate to control symptoms, other drugs are available on prescription from your doctor. If necessary, the doctor may prescribe combinations of a painkiller and domperidone, to promote better absorption of the painkillers as well as to control any nausea.

Some studies have demonstrated the efficacy of triptans in children, but most are still not recommended for patients under the age of 18 years. An exception is sumatriptan nasal spray, which can be given to adolescents aged over 12.

Preventing the attacks

The identification and management of trigger factors are the mainstay of migraine management in children. Non-drug treatments, such as biofeedback and relaxation techniques, are also very effective (see 'Living with migraine: complementary treatments', page 76).

It is rarely necessary to give daily preventive drugs to children. However, a short course may be necessary when the attacks are particularly disabling and are not controlled by symptomatic treatments. The most commonly prescribed preventive drugs for children are propranolol and pizotifen, with pizotifen being the drug of choice. Cyproheptadine has also been used with good results.

Headaches at school

It is always important to let the school know that your child has migraine, particularly as your child could develop an attack while at school. It is helpful to provide staff with specific written instructions for the management of your child's migraine, stressing the need for early treatment. However, schools have different rules regarding treatment. In some schools, teachers and/or nurses may agree to give some medication. In others, the school will telephone the carer (for example, parent) to collect the child if a migraine attack occurs.

Many parents and children are particularly worried that a migraine attack may interfere with important exams. Fortunately, migraine usually occurs after, rather than during, stress. This means that, although migraine may have disrupted studying for an exam, the child is usually unaffected on the day.

If frequent migraines affect your child's revision, or if several long exams are expected on consecutive days, other potential triggers should be avoided, by eating regularly, getting sufficient sleep, taking regular breaks, and getting fresh air and exercise. If necessary, a doctor can prescribe a short course of a beta blocker such as propranolol to help prevent attacks. Any drugs should be tested well in advance of any exams to ensure that side effects do not affect your child's performance.

Will they go away?

With time, boys tend to grow out of migraine, although the growth spurt at puberty can be a difficult time. Unfortunately, girls tend to grow into migraine, with many women noting a worsening of migraine in the years leading up to the menopause. Fortunately, both sexes usually find that migraine remits in later life.

Is it something more serious?

Few children have an underlying disorder causing their recurrent headaches, but if there is any cause for concern you should contact your doctor. Particular features that warrant medical advice include:

- an unaccountable increase in the frequency, severity or duration of the attacks
- recent school failure
- personality changes
- failure to grow or attain normal developmental goals
- fever
- persistent or progressive symptoms
- new symptoms.

When treatments fail

When children have frequent attacks of migraine or headache, and these are not controlled by simple management strategies, it is important to consider other causes.

Depression is often not recognised in children and should be considered in any child who has lost weight, become withdrawn and has disrupted sleep, when no physical cause for the symptoms can be found. Bullying at school or emotional upsets may be underlying factors that need addressing.

Children can also develop medication overuse headaches from the overuse of symptomatic drugs, even paracetamol (see 'Chronic daily headaches', page 124). To avoid this, symptomatic drugs should not be taken regularly on more than two to three days a week. If this problem does develop, the headache usually improves once all of the symptomatic drugs have been stopped.

KEY POINTS

■ Migraine attacks in children tend to be shorter than those in adults, and abdominal symptoms, such as nausea and vomiting, are often more pronounced than the headache

■ Inadequate nutrition (missed meals, too little fruit and vegetables) is probably the main trigger for migraine in children; other potential triggers include intensive sport, excitement, emotional upsets and, rarely, food intolerance or allergy

■ Junior ibuprofen is the drug of choice in treating migraine attacks in children

■ Parents should inform the school that their child is prone to migraine attacks

Headaches in elderly people

Reasons for headaches in elderly people

There are many reasons why elderly people experience headaches, including migraine, tension headaches and chronic daily headaches (see next chapter). Other headaches more specific to elderly people are discussed below.

Unless the cause is obvious and your headaches respond readily to treatment, you should check the likely causes with your doctor. He or she will be able to treat you or refer you for further tests or specialist treatment, as necessary.

Various causes
Brain tumours

It is unusual for headaches to be the first or only symptom of a brain tumour. More often, unusual weakness, visual loss or fits gradually progress as the tumour grows.

If you are over 50 when you experience an unusual headache that you have never had before, however, especially if it is associated with weakness or unpleasant sensations in your arm or leg, you should consult your doctor.

Carbon monoxide poisoning

During the winter, elderly people often use gas heaters, which may be faulty, burning inefficiently and emitting carbon monoxide. This can give rise to carbon monoxide poisoning, which is often missed as the true cause of a throbbing headache, fatigue (tiredness), dizziness and nausea.

A faulty gas fire or boiler burns with a yellow flame instead of a blue one and deposits soot on the ceramic plate behind it. If you suspect that your gas appliance is faulty, contact the Environmental Health Department.

Dental problems

Poor dentition and ill-fitting dentures can cause severe facial pain and trigger migraine attacks. Clicking or locking jaw joints can result in tension in the muscles that you use for chewing and eating, triggering pain in your temples.

If you suspect that this may be the problem, see your dentist, who may recommend simple exercises to relax your muscles, which can ease the pain. Drugs such as amitriptyline can also be helpful. Sometimes, referral to an orthodontic surgeon is necessary to adjust your bite.

Depression

Depression can result from a lack of sleep and poor nutrition and may be associated with headaches. Depression in elderly people can be difficult to treat, because many elderly people live alone with little social support to help combat loneliness.

Antidepressants, although often prescribed, should be used with care, because side effects are more common in older people.

Side effects of other medication

Medication taken for other health problems can cause headaches as a side effect, and this is often an unrecognised cause of headaches in elderly people. Drugs with the potential to trigger headaches include those used to treat certain heart conditions, such as nifedipine, glyceryl trinitrate and isosorbide dinitrate. Some drugs used for high blood pressure can worsen headaches, but others, such as beta blockers, can treat both.

If you take several different drugs for medical problems other than your headaches, check with your doctor or pharmacist to ensure that they are not a possible cause of your headaches.

Strokes

As people grow older, their arteries fur up like a kettle, narrowing the blood vessels and reducing the blood flow. This is known as atherosclerosis and is linked to an increased risk of strokes and heart attacks.

Occasionally, migraine can mimic symptoms (such as visual disturbances) of mini-strokes, known as transient ischaemic attacks or TIAs. This is unlikely in migraineurs who have experienced the same migraine attacks throughout their lives, but may be important in those who develop migraine for the first time in later life. Anyone who develops problems with vision for the first time should consult their doctor without delay.

Temporal arteritis

Temporal arteritis is rare in young people, usually affecting those over the age of 50, particularly women. Its cause is unknown. The arteries in the temples and elsewhere become inflamed and swollen. The arteries beneath the skin of the temples become painful, particularly when touched, and the skin over the artery becomes red. A headache is also a symptom, the pain being on one or both sides and worse over the affected blood vessels. Sometimes, chewing causes pain in the muscles of the jaw.

The disorder may affect other blood vessels inside the head, including the temporal artery, which supplies the eye. If this happens, blindness may result. If you suspect that you may have temporal arteritis, it is vital that you seek medical advice as an emergency early on to prevent blindness.

Your doctor can do a simple blood test to help confirm the diagnosis, although it is occasionally necessary to take a small sample of the affected blood vessel. Steroids rapidly ease the pain and prevent blindness developing, but the treatment needs to be continued for a long time.

Trigeminal neuralgia

Trigeminal neuralgia is more common in elderly people, affecting slightly more women than men. The pain is restricted to a nerve in the face, which causes sudden spasms of severe shooting pain (in the cheek and jaw) lasting for only a few seconds – this is often described as being like an electric shock. The pain occurs in bouts every day for several weeks or months.

Triggers include chewing, cleaning your teeth, shaving and cold wind on your face. It is usually controlled with the drug carbamazepine. A few sufferers continue to have unremitting pain and may need surgical treatment.

KEY POINTS

■ Headaches in older people may have an underlying cause that needs specialist treatment

■ It is unusual for headaches to be the first or only symptom of a brain tumour

■ Dental problems can cause severe facial pain and trigger migraine

■ Headaches may be a side effect of prescription medications, such as some heart drugs

■ Temporal arteritis can cause headaches and needs to be diagnosed and treated early, before it causes blindness

Chronic daily headaches

What type of headache is it?

The most common causes of daily headaches are those resulting from muscle contraction or related to stress or tension. Both are described below. Migraine does not occur daily, but attacks can be present in people also suffering from daily headaches, which can lead to confusion about the diagnosis. When several types of headaches occur, it is very important that each headache is diagnosed separately.

Treating the cause of the headaches

It is more important to treat the cause of your daily headaches before tackling your migraine because migraine often improves without further intervention. Daily headaches can result from over-frequent use of symptomatic treatments – often causing the headaches to become unresponsive to all other treatment strategies.

Daily headaches may be a symptom of an underlying disease – for example, temporal arteritis (see page 122) – or a chronic infection – for example, sinusitis (see page 145). If the underlying disease is treated, the headaches often resolve. Less frequently, daily headaches have no clear underlying cause and respond poorly to any treatments tried. Once serious underlying causes have been excluded, you can be helped to cope with the pain.

Muscle-contraction headaches

Most people have experienced the pain of aching muscles after unaccustomed exercise. Your muscles may feel sore and tender to the touch, and gentle massage or lying in a hot bath often helps. The muscles of your head are no different. Often the pain is localised and you can point to the site of the pain, in contrast to the generalised pain of 'tension' headaches (see below).

The pain can arise some distance from where it is actually felt in the head: pain in your temples may originate from your jaw joints; neck and shoulder muscle pains can also cause headaches. Although painkillers may provide temporary relief within 30 to 45 minutes, they are treating only the symptoms and not the cause.

Effective management should be directed at treating and preventing the underlying physical problem using treatments such as exercise, physiotherapy, massage, etc. Obvious causes, such as cradling a telephone on your shoulder for long periods at work or sitting at a computer stationed at the wrong height, can often be rectified very easily. (For more details, see 'Other causes of headaches', page 140.)

Stress-related tension headaches

Psychological stress or anxiety may cause the muscles in the scalp and neck to become tense, resulting in a headache – sufferers often describe this type of tension headache as a 'band around my head' or 'a weight pressing down on top of my head'. The pain is often all over your head and is present most of the time, waxing and waning through the day. It may interfere with your sleep, particularly if you are depressed or anxious.

Painkillers typically have little effect, although they may dull the pain for a couple of hours or so. If your headache is to be managed effectively, the underlying cause must be treated – for example, dealing with any depression, managing stress, etc. (see *Understanding Stress*, *Understanding Depression* – titles in the Family Doctor series). If necessary, you may find a course of antidepressants, such as amitriptyline, useful, particularly if your sleep is affected.

Medication overuse headaches

The limited use of symptomatic drugs, such as painkillers, triptans or ergotamine, is safe and effective. However, the frequent use of these drugs for headaches can have the opposite effect.

Taking painkillers too regularly can perpetuate the cycle of pain rather than relieve it and may lead to headaches occurring on most days, sometimes daily, often with more frequent migraine attacks as well.

What are the symptoms?

Typically, you may have experienced infrequent attacks of migraine that you have controlled with simple painkillers or specific symptomatic migraine treatments. For varying reasons, you may have increased the use of your medication until you are taking it on most days, sometimes several times a day.

This may be because an additional headache has developed, perhaps as a result of stress or muscular

Headache caused by muscular tension in the head

Tension in the muscles of your head, neck and shoulders can cause headaches. Often the cause of the pain can arise some distance from where it is felt in the head. Effective treatment is directed at the underlying physical problem, not at relief of the symptoms.

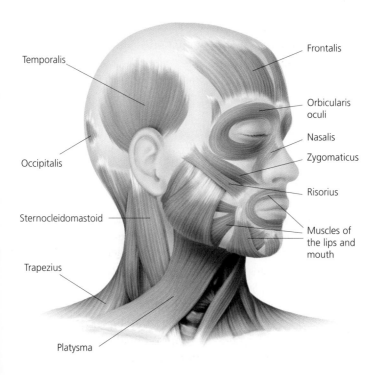

Temporalis

Frontalis

Orbicularis oculi

Nasalis

Zygomaticus

Occipitalis

Risorius

Sternocleidomastoid

Muscles of the lips and mouth

Trapezius

Platysma

pain, or your fear of a migraine getting out of hand has led to pre-emptive treatment. Gradually, your headaches increase in frequency until they occur on most days.

Your daily headache is usually worse on waking, perhaps because your blood levels of the painkillers are at their lowest at this time of day. The pain is dull and constant but may fluctuate throughout the day. It is temporarily relieved (but in many cases only partially) with painkillers or migraine treatments.

Despite this lack of treatment effect, you may find that a migraine develops unless you take a treatment, continuing the cycle of medication overuse. Other symptoms include fatigue, nausea, irritability, memory loss and difficulty sleeping.

How does medication overuse headache occur?

Medication overuse headache may occur in anyone who takes symptomatic headache treatments regularly on more than three days a week for three or more months. It makes no difference how much you take – if you regularly use the full dose of painkillers on less than a couple of days a week, you are unlikely to develop daily headaches. However, if you take just a couple of painkillers (that is, less than the full dose) on most days, you may be making your headaches worse.

The exact mechanism of this type of headache is unknown, but it is generally believed that a disturbance of central pain systems is involved. Interestingly, only those people who are prone to headaches seem to develop this syndrome, and it is not often seen in people who take daily painkillers for reasons other than headache, such as arthritis or back pain.

How is it treated?

The headaches are resistant to most medication, and the only effective treatment is to stop the drugs – either immediately or by gradually reducing the amount over several weeks. Withdrawal symptoms consisting of excruciating headaches, nausea, vomiting, anxiety and insomnia appear within 48 hours, and may last for up to two weeks.

Clinical studies show that up to 60 per cent of sufferers who are weaned off the drugs improve, although it can take up to three months before full improvement is seen. A doctor can prescribe drugs such as amitriptyline and naproxen (to be taken every day) to help withdrawal. However, these drugs are effective only if all other headache medication is stopped. Even if the headaches do remain three months after stopping the drugs, the underlying cause usually becomes apparent and is more responsive to specific treatment.

KEY POINTS

- Chronic daily headache is often caused by muscle contraction or is related to stress

- Daily headaches may have an underlying cause, such as sinusitis

- Taking painkillers too regularly, usually on more than three days a week for three or more months, can also lead to daily headaches (medication overuse headache)

Cluster headache and chronic paroxysmal hemicrania

What are these headaches?

Cluster headache and chronic paroxysmal hemicrania (CPH) are related headaches that are quite different from migraine. The attacks are short-lasting compared with migraine attacks, and follow a typical pattern of symptoms.

Although the symptoms are so specific that the diagnosis is obvious once recognised, their rarity means that they may be misdiagnosed as migraine or another type of headache, particularly if the sufferer also has migraine. Many sufferers do not get the right treatment for several years. Although there is rarely an identifiable underlying cause, and no specific tests are necessary to confirm the diagnosis, some cases, particularly those with atypical (not conforming to type) symptoms, may be the result of other causes.

Cluster headache

Cluster headache is an excruciatingly painful headache. It affects about 1 in 1,000 people, and is five times more common among men than women.

The condition has been known by many different names over the centuries, including migrainous neuralgia, Horton's headache and histamine headache. The pattern of cluster headache is very typical.

The headaches usually begin to appear during the late 20s or early 30s. There seems to be some link with smoking because many sufferers are heavy smokers, either currently or in the past. Those who have never smoked will often say that their parents smoked heavily. Unfortunately, stopping smoking makes little difference to the symptoms.

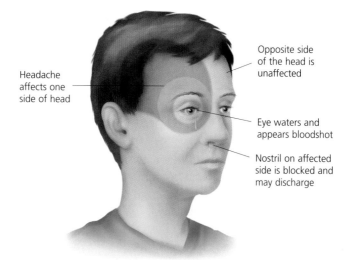

Headache affects one side of head

Opposite side of the head is unaffected

Eye waters and appears bloodshot

Nostril on affected side is blocked and may discharge

Cluster headache is an excruciatingly painful headache that is five times more common among men than women. The headache always occurs on the same side during each cluster and is usually centred over one eye.

As the name suggests, the attacks come in clusters, typically for several weeks once or twice a year at the same time of year. A few sufferers have chronic cluster headache with very little remission from attacks.

During a cluster period, sufferers experience an average of one to three attacks each day of very severe one-sided pain lasting between 20 minutes and 2 to 3 hours. The attacks often wake the sufferer from sleep at a similar time every night. The pain builds up rapidly to peak within a few minutes of its onset.

The headache always occurs on the same side during each cluster and is usually centred over one eye, which waters and appears bloodshot. The nostril on the affected side feels blocked and there may be a discharge. The opposite side of the head is completely unaffected.

Unlike migraine, which is aggravated by movement, cluster headache sufferers will often pace up and down, holding their head, rocking it back and forth. They may put so much pressure on the painful area or rub it so hard that it bleeds. Many sufferers will go to a window or go outside to get some fresh air. The pain is so severe and intense that some sufferers become aggressive during an attack or repeatedly hit their heads. Those who have experienced other painful conditions, such as kidney stones, say that the pain of cluster headache is much worse. The symptoms subside rapidly, but the area around the affected eye may feel 'bruised' between attacks.

Alcohol may trigger attacks but only during the cluster. Alcohol and other substances that dilate blood vessels, such as glyceryl trinitrate and histamine, have been used in research to provoke attacks. No other triggers have been identified and avoiding migraine triggers is irrelevant, although a few sufferers have reported a link with times of particular stress.

What causes cluster headache?

Despite intense medical research, the cause remains elusive. Much interest centres on the timing of the attacks, which appears to be linked to circadian rhythms (the biological or 'body' clock). Many sufferers report that their clusters are more likely to start around spring and autumn.

Recent research has highlighted changes in part of the brain called the hypothalamus, the area that controls the body clock.

Will I have it forever?

Fortunately for many sufferers, particularly those with chronic cluster headache, cluster headache does seem to improve in later life (after the age of 50).

Treatment of cluster headache

Apart from avoiding alcohol during clusters to prevent attacks the main treatment of cluster headache involves taking medication. The treatment may be acute, aimed at treating the symptoms when they start, or prophylactic, which involves taking drugs every day to try to prevent attacks developing.

Most sufferers need both acute and prophylactic drugs to control attacks during a cluster, because prophylactic drugs are rarely completely effective.

Acute (symptomatic) treatment

For many sufferers, inhaling 100 per cent oxygen, via a facial mask, is safe and effective. Oxygen should be inhaled for 10 to 20 minutes at 7 litres per minute, while in a sitting position, leaning forward.

From 1 February 2006, new regulations for home oxygen prescribing delivery came into force. Whereas before, sufferers obtained their oxygen through pharmacies from a prescription from their GP, now the GP sends a Home Oxygen Order Form to the oxygen supplier that has won the contract for each particular region. The supplier then delivers the oxygen cylinders direct to the person's door.

All cylinders will come complete with their own integral high regulator of up to 15 litres per minute. The oxygen supplier will also provide non-rebreathing masks. Static 1,360-litre cylinders and ambulatory 460-litre cylinders, for portable use, are available.

Your doctor may prescribe injections of six milligrams of sumatriptan, given under your skin, which can be used when a cluster starts, and this gives benefit in less than ten minutes. A maximum of two injections in 24 hours is recommended. The side effects and contraindications are the same as for migraine (see 'Living with migraine: seeing a doctor', page 58).

Prophylactic (preventive) treatment

Drugs taken daily can reduce the frequency and severity of your attacks, making them more responsive to acute treatment. Prophylactic drugs seem to be more effective the earlier they are started in a cluster period. If they do not seem to be working, it may be that the dose is inadequate or you need a different drug.

You should continue the treatment for the usual duration of the cluster, then reduce the dose gradually over one to two weeks. If attacks break through, increase the dose until you have maintained control and then reduce it every couple of weeks until the cluster is over.

It is common for drugs to be combined to enhance their effectiveness. Drugs known as calcium channel blockers (which relax the muscle in blood vessels), such as verapamil, are usually tried first. The starting dose is low but is increased over seven to ten days. A few people need to take higher doses under close medical supervision. The most common side effect is constipation, but dizziness, fatigue and nausea may also occur.

Ergotamine can be used daily for episodic cluster headache. It should not be used regularly for chronic cluster headache, because it can cause long-term problems, constricting the blood supply to small blood vessels, particularly those in your fingers and toes. The drug is given as a suppository one to four hours before an expected attack, for example, at bedtime for night-time attacks. This strategy should be continued only for the expected duration of the cluster and for no longer than six to eight weeks.

Corticosteroids, such as prednisolone, taken by mouth can be effective at preventing a cluster if they are started early.

Methysergide (which is chemically related to ergotamine) is taken by mouth and is one of the most effective prophylactic drugs, although its long-term use has been associated with the development of scar tissue at the back of the abdomen, which can interfere with the urinary system. This complication is known as retroperitoneal fibrosis, but it is rare and has not been known to occur if a one-month drug 'holiday' is taken for every six months of use. Side effects of nausea, diarrhoea and muscle cramps are common, but are less likely to occur if the dose is increased slowly.

Lithium (a mineral that affects the blood chemistry) is often used in chronic cluster headache. You will need regular blood tests to make sure that the level in your bloodstream is adequate. Side effects include mild nausea, weakness and thirst, which usually wear off with continued use. Diuretic drugs (which increase the output of urine) should not be taken with lithium because they can enhance the levels of lithium in your bloodstream and result in toxic doses.

Pizotifen (a serotonin antagonist) and sodium valproate (an anticonvulsant) have been recommended by some authorities, but there is only limited evidence for their effectiveness in the treatment of cluster headache.

Surgery
Several surgical strategies have been tried, including steroid injections into the occipital nerve at the back of the head on the affected side, but this usually gives only brief respite.

If a person's symptoms are completely resistant to all other treatments, surgery of the trigeminal ganglion (a nerve junction box behind the cheek) has been advocated, although this is not without risks (interfering with sensation in the face and mouth) and cannot be guaranteed to be effective.

Chronic paroxysmal hemicrania
Chronic paroxysmal hemicrania (CPH) is also rare. Unlike cluster headache, it affects two to three times more women than men and usually starts in the early 30s. Attacks follow a typical pattern of brief attacks of excruciating one-sided pain, lasting for just a few minutes, occurring between 5 and 40 times a day.

Unlike with cluster headache, CPH sufferers prefer to sit quietly or even curl up in a ball in bed during attacks. Most sufferers notice that their eye on the affected side waters and reddens.

The cause of CPH is unknown, but the condition almost invariably responds to the anti-inflammatory drug indometacin – as a prophylactic treatment. Triggers include bending or turning the head and hormonal changes, such as those that occur with menstruation.

As with cluster headache, verapamil has also been used with beneficial effects. Drugs do not affect the tendency of the condition to fluctuate. A few sufferers need life-long therapy, but most will have periods of remission, which can last for several years.

KEY POINTS

■ Cluster headaches come in episodes lasting several weeks with attacks usually occurring once or twice a year

■ Acute therapy (for example, 100 per cent oxygen) can be used to treat cluster headaches, while prophylactic drugs may help to prevent attacks

■ Chronic paroxysmal hemicrania (CPH) causes brief attacks of severe one-sided pain lasting for just a few minutes between 5 and 40 times a day; the attacks can be prevented with drugs

Other causes
of headaches

Other types of headaches
The most common headaches, muscle-contraction and
tension headaches, have been described earlier (see
page 125). This chapter describes another dozen or so
causes of headaches and their management.

Stress-related (tension) headaches
These band-like headaches are the result of increased
tension in the muscles of the scalp and neck. They
typically occur at times of emotional upset, such as
crying, and are usually short lasting as the trigger
resolves, without the need for drugs. However, long
periods of stress or depression can result in daily
headaches requiring specific intervention (see 'Chronic
daily headaches', page 124).

Hangovers
Few people are fortunate enough never to have
experienced a hangover. Obviously, the best way to
avoid a hangover is not to drink, but here are five
'rules' to help minimise the effects of alcohol.

1. Never drink on an empty stomach

Try to 'line' your stomach by eating something before drinking, preferably a fatty food, to slow down the rate at which alcohol reaches your bloodstream.

2. Don't mix your drinks

Some drinks contain chemicals called congeners, which have been implicated in contributing to hangovers – these are small molecules produced during the fermentation and distillation of certain alcohols, for example, brandy and bourbon. Vodka and gin are low in congeners and are less likely to cause a hangover.

3. Mix alcohol with fruit juice

There is some evidence that the natural sugar fructose helps to speed up the metabolism (breakdown) of alcohol so there is less chance of having a hangover. Fructose is found in fruit, fruit juice and honey. Stick to drinks mixed with fruit juices, and drink a large glass of fruit juice before going to bed.

4. Drink slowly

Your body eventually turns alcohol into carbon dioxide and water, but first alcohol is broken down in your liver to acetaldehyde and acetic acid. Your body can break down alcohol at the rate of approximately one unit per hour, equivalent to half a pint of beer, one standard measure of spirits or one glass of wine. If you drink faster than this, too much acetaldehyde builds up and this chemical may be responsible for the hangover.

Alternating an alcoholic drink with a soft drink is a good idea, or dilute your drinks with fruit juice or mixers. However, be warned that research has shown that fizzy mixers cause alcohol to reach your bloodstream faster than still mixers – that is, you'll get drunk faster on scotch and soda than scotch and water.

5. Use survival strategies when you get home

Drink a large glass of fruit juice and lots of water before you go to bed to counteract the dehydrating effects of alcohol. Avoid black coffee; there is little evidence that it counteracts the effects of alcohol and it may upset your stomach more because, like alcohol, it also irritates the lining of your stomach. Eat something to counteract the effects of the alcohol, but keep the snack light and easy to digest, such as toast and honey. Take a couple of soluble pain-killers as well. Half to one teaspoon of baking soda in half a cup of tepid water can help settle your stomach.

Head injury

Most people complain of a headache after a head injury where the injury is relatively mild and they have not lost consciousness. The headache usually disappears after a few hours or days. However mild the injury, it is important to rest, preferably lying flat in bed, until the headache has gone. Simple painkillers such as aspirin or paracetamol can be taken.

When the injury is more severe and the patient has been unconscious, even for a short time, you must consult a doctor. The patient may be admitted to hospital overnight, because occasionally bleeding inside the head may occur, forming a clot. This causes further symptoms, such as slowing of the pulse, drowsiness or unconsciousness. Surgical treatment is necessary to remove the blood clot.

Sports headaches

Sport can also trigger attacks, particularly when the exercise is intense and sustained. The simplest strategy for prevention is to maintain blood glucose levels with glucose sweets, drink plenty of fluids to avoid dehydration, and take exercise gradually and progressively where possible.

Minor blows to your head during sport, such as heading a football or a hit on your face in a rugby tackle, can trigger an instantaneous migraine aura, not always followed by a headache. Although you should seek medical advice, these attacks have been shown to be benign (non-serious).

Weekend headaches

Obviously, hangovers are more common at weekends but, irrespective of how much you have had to drink, you may notice that if you sleep in at weekends you develop a generalised headache. This may be because of the extra sleep, but could also be the result of having a delayed breakfast or even caffeine withdrawal.

Migraine is also more likely to occur at a weekend, particularly if you have a regular working week from Monday to Friday. This pattern is most likely to arise from a combination of triggers building up during the working week, such as stress, a lack of sleep and missed meals. This is then compounded by the additional weekend triggers of relaxation after a stressful week, sleeping in and a delayed breakfast. Keeping a daily trigger diary can help (see 'Living with migraine: self-help', page 42), but you may need to follow a stricter routine at weekends, getting up and eating breakfast nearer to your usual time.

Headaches during sex (coital headaches)

Headaches associated with sexual activity affect men more than women and are more common in people who have migraine or high blood pressure. There is also a link with exercise headaches.

The most common symptom is a dull headache at the back of your head, which gradually intensifies as sexual excitement increases. It is thought to be related to excessive muscular contraction of your head and neck.

The headache can be prevented by deliberately relaxing your muscles, although, if this is not effective, an anti-inflammatory drug (such as naproxen) or the beta blocker propranolol can be prescribed by your doctor. Some people experience a sudden severe explosive headache at orgasm, also known as 'thunderclap headache', that lasts for 20 to 30 minutes.

Although coital headaches rarely have a serious underlying cause, they can sometimes result from bleeding in the brain. You should, therefore, seek medical advice if you experience these headaches, because tests may be necessary to rule out such a cause.

Eyestrain

Weakness or imbalance of your eye muscles, or errors in the focusing power of your eye, may occasionally cause headaches. The headache develops and increases in severity when your eyes are strained, resulting in discomfort and a feeling of heaviness around your eyes.

Wearing glasses or contact lenses can often correct the underlying problem and should therefore improve this type of headache, so have your eyes tested.

Sinusitis

Sinusitis is generally a short-lasting infection (acute sinusitis) associated with a generalised headache, fever and pain localised to the affected sinus (an air-filled pocket in bones surrounding your nose, cheeks and eyes). The pain is made worse by jolting or sudden movements and by bending over. There may be tenderness over the affected sinus and sometimes a slight swelling of your lower eyelid.

A vague discomfort in your forehead, between your eyes and across your nose, can be caused by a continuing infection, resulting in chronic sinusitis. Sinusitis is usually treated with antibiotics and decongestants.

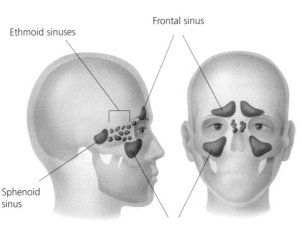

Ethmoid sinuses

Frontal sinus

Sphenoid sinus

Maxillary sinus

The sinuses are several air-filled cavities located in the skull bones around the eyes, cheeks and nose. An infection in the sinuses can cause pain in the infected sinus, fever and a headache.

Dental problems

A headache can be a symptom of an infection in your mouth, which may be associated with a low-grade fever. A clicking jaw, teeth grinding or clenching can also result in a headache, usually associated with tenderness in your jaw joint and the affected muscles. A visit to your dentist can confirm the problem.

You may need to use a mouth guard or may be referred to an orthodontist for more specific treatment. Relaxation exercises can help headaches associated with teeth grinding or clenching because these problems are often made worse by stress. Headaches can also result from chewing gum – an easy cause to resolve!

Cervical spondylosis

Cervical spondylosis is a degenerative condition of the bones of the neck, possibly causing compression of the spinal cord. Most people over the age of 40 have some cervical spondylosis in their spine and these changes can be seen on an X-ray.

In most people, this does not cause any symptoms, but occasionally changes in the upper part of your cervical spine may cause pain starting in the back of your neck extending up the back of your head. However, muscular pain arising from your neck and shoulder muscles is a more common cause of headache than spinal problems.

Neck injury

The most common neck injury is known as 'whiplash', which typically follows a car crash. In this type of accident, your neck first over-extends backwards and then over-flexes forwards. You may notice tenderness in your neck soon after the accident, but this then

How whiplash is caused

The most frequent cause of whiplash injury is a motor vehicle accident.

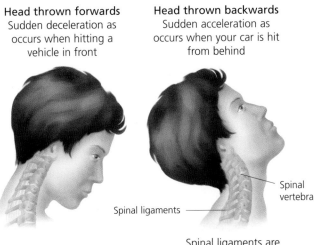

Head thrown forwards
Sudden deceleration as occurs when hitting a vehicle in front

Head thrown backwards
Sudden acceleration as occurs when your car is hit from behind

Spinal vertebra

Spinal ligaments

Spinal ligaments are overstretched

develops into more generalised neck and head pains made worse by neck movement.

These pains usually settle over a couple of weeks, but occasionally persist, developing into 'whiplash syndrome'. Generalised headache is worse on waking and is exacerbated by physical or mental exertion. Although some neck movements aggravate the pain, others ease it. Some people feel dizzy and experience noises in their ears, throat discomfort, impaired memory and concentration, and fatigue.

The treatment is rest, painkillers, a neck collar and physiotherapy. Many people wear the collar for too long, which prevents their neck muscles from regaining their strength – necessary for complete recovery.

High blood pressure

It is common for blood pressure to increase with advancing years and no cause for this is usually found. In most cases, moderately raised blood pressure does not cause headaches. However, very high blood pressure can cause headaches, which improve when your blood pressure is lowered.

If your headache results from high blood pressure, you would usually feel it at the back of your head, it would be present on waking and it would be pulsating or throbbing in nature. You can self-monitor your blood pressure at home, although this should be done in consultation with your doctor, who can prescribe medication to lower your blood pressure if appropriate.

Brain tumours

Headaches are rarely the first sign of a brain tumour. In addition, the symptoms of the brain tumour usually develop gradually and become progressively worse, unlike the episodic nature of migraine, which is associated with complete freedom from symptoms between attacks.

If there is any sudden change in the pattern or duration of your usual headaches, or if new symptoms occur, you should see your doctor.

KEY POINTS

- Headaches can result from stiff and painful muscles, especially in your scalp, jaw, neck, shoulders and upper back

- Headaches may be related to stress or may accompany a hangover

- Sometimes headaches follow a sporting injury or a head injury

- Some people are prone to headaches at weekends, possibly as a result of a change in routine

- Headaches may also be caused by eye problems, dental problems, sinusitis, spinal problems or high blood pressure

- Headaches are rarely a sign of a brain tumour

Questions
and answers

Does migraine cause any long-term damage?
There is no firm evidence to suggest that frequent
attacks of migraine cause any permanent damage to
your brain. Migraineurs are usually fit and well
between attacks, unless they have other specific
medical or psychiatric problems. Some doctors even
argue that migraine may be protective, by forcing you
to withdraw from a build-up of stimuli that could
otherwise be potentially harmful to your health.

Is it true that people with migraine are more likely to
have a stroke?
The majority of studies suggest that stroke is very
slightly more likely to occur in young migraineurs, but
the absolute risk is very small, with stroke affecting
fewer than 6 in 100,000 women at the age of 20. The
problem with studying a link between stroke and
migraine is that stroke is very rare in the age group
that suffers the most migraines.

However, certain risk factors, such as smoking,
particularly in women who also take the combined oral

contraceptive pill, may slightly increase the risk of stroke. The risk of stroke as a result of smoking is much greater than the risk as a result of migraine.

Why doesn't my doctor send me for any tests to diagnose migraine?
There are no tests that can confirm migraine. Migraine is usually diagnosed from the description of your attacks. If your attacks are typical of migraine, and an examination is normal, you won't need any further investigations.

I'd like to get fit but every time I start an exercise programme, I wake up the next day with a migraine. What can I do?
Studies show that fit people are less likely to have problems with migraine. Regular exercise has many benefits for your body and mind. Unfortunately, getting fit can make things worse before they get better. Strenuous infrequent exercise causes stiff, aching muscles and may trigger migraine attacks. However, this is no reason to avoid exercise.

You can prevent unnecessary pain if you exercise regularly and at the right intensity for your initial fitness level. Stretching exercises at the beginning and end of a workout can ease muscle tension, as can a hot bath or sauna. Deep heat creams or heat pads are also useful.

Many people start an exercise programme at the same time as a new diet, and this can act as an additional trigger. It is important to eat sensibly and not to 'crash' diet.

I travel a lot for work but find that long plane trips inevitably trigger migraine. What can I do?

Travelling is a common trigger for migraine for several reasons. First, there is the stress of preparing for a trip – clearing your desk at work, tidying your house, packing, etc. Then there is the stress of travelling – carrying heavy suitcases, missing meals, coping with a lack of sleep and jet-lag, climate changes, etc.

Flying is associated with specific problems of reduced oxygen in the circulating air, dehydration, erratic mealtimes and sitting in a cramped seat for several hours. Advance planning can help. Take some snacks to eat, avoid alcohol, drink plenty of fluids (carry a bottle of still mineral water with you) and walk around the plane regularly.

I suffer from two or three migraines every week. Could I have 'cluster migraine'?

Although the term 'cluster migraine' is sometimes used, it is meaningless because it confuses two quite separate conditions: migraine and cluster headache. Migraine is an episodic headache with complete freedom from symptoms between attacks. The symptoms last for about one to three days. The frequency of attacks varies, but may average one attack every two to eight weeks. Cluster headache is much rarer and is very different. Attacks may occur daily, often at night, for several weeks. The headaches last between one and two hours, always affecting the same side of your head.

The distinction is important, because the treatment for each condition is quite different. People who report several 'migraines' each week often have a new additional headache as well as their usual migraine. In these cases, the different headaches need to be diagnosed correctly so that effective treatment can be given.

I've been using a triptan for several years and it is very effective. The leaflet that comes with the tablets says I shouldn't take it if I'm over 65. Will I have to stop taking it?

Triptans constrict the blood vessels in your head that become dilated in migraine, hence their effect. However, the concern is that diseased blood vessels, such as those in the heart, could also be affected. This is not a problem for young, fit, healthy people.

The concern is that, as people age, their blood vessels fur up, like a kettle. This is known as atherosclerosis and increases the risk of heart disease and a stroke by narrowing the blood vessels. Drugs that further narrow blood vessels should be avoided. Obviously, some people are more at risk of atherosclerosis than others, but it is not always easy to identify who may be affected. Therefore, there is a general recommendation that older people should avoid taking triptans.

I don't understand why my doctor says that I shouldn't take painkillers every day, telling me it's giving me headaches, and then prescribes a different medication for me to take every day.

Symptomatic drugs should be used infrequently, on no more than two or three days a week, to treat the symptoms of migraine or headaches. It is now recognised that if you take symptomatic treatments, such as painkillers or triptans, on most days, this can be linked to daily headache, which improves only when you stop taking the drugs.

If your headaches are frequent, you will be prescribed a very different type of medication to take every day to prevent, rather than treat, attacks. These drugs work in a different way to help stop the attacks developing.

I only used to get migraine once every couple of months but over the last year the attacks have been getting more frequent. I now get them every day and nothing seems to help. Can I have something stronger to take?

Daily headaches are not the same as migraine and should not be treated as such. In addition, taking drugs to control your symptoms does not treat the cause and may make your condition worse. Stronger medication is not appropriate.

Once the serious causes of headaches have been excluded, you should stop taking daily painkillers. This, in itself, may improve your headache. Any remaining headaches can be diagnosed and then treated correctly.

How long will I have to keep taking tablets every day to prevent migraine? Will I have to take them for the rest of my life?

Most preventive drugs for migraine are taken only for a few months to break the cycle of frequent attacks. This is usually adequate, although, if the attacks return as the dose is reduced, it may be necessary to return to the original dose for a further few months.

If you take the drugs for too long, side effects can build up and create additional problems. This may be why stopping preventive drugs is also associated with improvement! You may need to repeat courses of preventive drugs if the attacks become more frequent, however.

I'm not depressed but my doctor has prescribed antidepressants for my migraine. Why?
Few drugs used in migraine are exclusive to migraine. Antidepressants, particularly amitriptyline, are commonly used to prevent migraine attacks. They have an effect on serotonin, a chemical found in your brain that has been implicated in migraine as well as in depression. Therefore, even if you are not depressed, these drugs can be very effective.

My blood pressure is normal but my doctor has prescribed the same drug that my mother takes for her high blood pressure. Why?
Several research studies have shown that certain drugs used to treat high blood pressure also effectively prevent migraine. The reason why these drugs are effective for migraine is not known. It is unlikely that it is anything to do with their effect on blood pressure, because the doses used in migraine are much lower than those needed to treat high blood pressure.

Is there a genetic cause of migraine?
It is generally thought that migraine can run in families, typically from mother to daughter. Researchers have looked for a genetic link by studying identical twins, who have exactly the same genes. If inherited genes are the only cause of migraine, either identical twins should both have migraine or neither of them should have migraine. Studies show that this is not

always the case, suggesting that environmental factors, such as how you respond to potential triggers etc., also play an important role. Migraine is such a common condition that it is highly likely that at least one other member of a family will have migraine without it being an inherited condition.

How to help the migraine clinic doctor help you

Before you arrive

It is a great help if you have made a few notes. Keep a record of your headaches in a diary for several weeks, noting the time that your headaches start, how long they last, your other symptoms and the dates of your menstrual periods, if you think that they are related.

Medical history

Your doctor will first need to decide what type of headache you have. To help answer this, he or she will need to know roughly how old you were when your headaches first started, how often you get them, how long they last and what your symptoms are. This information helps the doctor to build up a picture of your headaches. This is important because there are no specific tests for migraine, or the majority of other headaches, so the diagnosis is based mainly on your own description.

If your doctor decides that you probably do have migraine, he or she will be looking for ways to help you cope. You will be asked about remedies that you have already tried, and it is helpful if you have written these down, otherwise there is bound to be something that you forget! Make notes about changes that you have made to your lifestyle and whether or not these have worked, about stress and sleep and other trigger factors, about the tablets, suppositories, inhalers or injections, about the doctors, physiotherapist, chiropractors, osteopaths, herbalists, homoeopaths and hypnotists, and so the list goes on!

Your doctor will also ask you about your general well-being and past illnesses.

Treatment and advice

If you have migraine, and only migraine, then this will be obvious by this stage of the consultation; if you have a mixture of headaches, or if the description of your headaches does not suggest any immediate diagnosis, however, you may need to keep a detailed record of your symptoms for several weeks before your follow-up appointment. This should help your doctor to make a diagnosis.

There is no cure for migraine – this is a hard but undeniable fact of life. Fortunately, however, there is a lot that can be done to improve your symptoms by reducing the number of attacks and finding more effective treatments. The details of migraine management will depend on your particular needs, but generally the first step towards reducing the number of migraines is to identify your trigger factors.

If these simple measures do not bring about an improvement, your doctor will discuss with you the option of taking daily preventive drugs. Medication to treat the actual attacks will also be discussed. At the end of the consultation, your clinic doctor will write to the GP who referred you with a summary and suggestions about management.

You will usually be invited to return within three months, but this depends on the frequency of your attacks and your individual case.

Follow-up visits

It is not always possible to make a diagnosis at your first visit. Over a series of visits, and with the help of a diary card, your doctor can give you further advice and, if necessary, adjust your treatment. Alternatively, if you do not have migraine you may be referred to a centre that deals with your particular type of headache.

After a few visits, all being well, many patients find that they do not need to return to the clinic because they are much improved. They are pleased to know that they can be referred back should the need arise – the patients and the doctors hope that it does not.

Your ideas

The doctors at the clinic are always interested to hear any worries that you may have about your headaches. Do not be embarrassed about this because a few words of explanation now can save a lot of worry later on. Any ideas that you have can help our research and further our understanding of headaches.

Research and publications

Medical staff at the clinic undertake research projects; their results and findings are published in the medical press. An independent Ethics Committee has assessed all clinical trials before they start. No patients are included in trials unless they have given their full written permission and have been fully informed about what participation in the study involves.

They are also free to withdraw from a study at any time. Involvement in research projects does not affect your routine medical care, although it often allows early access to new treatments.

Useful information

We have included the following organisations because, on preliminary investigation, they may be of use to the reader. However, we do not have first-hand experience of each organisation and so cannot guarantee the organisation's integrity. The reader must therefore exercise his or her own discretion and judgement when making further enquiries.

Migraine organisations in the UK

The City of London Migraine Clinic
22 Charterhouse Square
London EC1M 6DX
Tel: 020 7251 3322
Fax: 020 7490 2183
Website: www.colmc.org.uk

A medical charity working with St Bartholomew's Hospital in London. Dr Marcia Wilkinson, the Clinic's Patron and Dr Nat Blau, Medical Director and Consultant Neurologist, founded the Clinic, in its present guise, in 1980.

Who can be seen?

People living and working in the UK should ask for a letter of referral from their GP. There is no charge for referring patients. The patients come mostly from London and the Home Counties, but the clinic does see patients from all over the UK and even from all over the world.

How they raise money?

As a charity, there is no charge for anyone who is entitled to NHS treatment, although the clinic hopes that all the patients will be kind enough to make a generous donation to support its research and keep the service going. People not eligible for the NHS treatment, including those from abroad, can be seen as private patients – a referral letter is still required.

Doctors donate all fees from patients to the clinic. The clinic does not receive any government support or grants, so they are always grateful for donations and particularly covenants. When the clinic first started, patients' donations covered one-third of running costs. With rising overheads, this figure has been reduced to one-tenth, so all donations are gratefully received.

Migraine Action Association

Unit 6, Oakley Hay Lodge Business Park, Great Folds Road Great Oakley, Northants NN18 9AS
Tel: 01536 461333
Fax: 01536 461444
Helpline: 0870 050 5898
Email: info@migraine.org.uk
Website: www.migraine.org.uk

Supports research, offers information on the understanding and treatment of migraine and has local self-help groups.

Migraine Trust

2nd Floor, 55–56 Russell Square
London WC1B 4HP
Tel: 020 7436 1336
Fax: 020 7436 2880
Helpline: 020 7462 6601
Email: info@migrainetrust.org
Website: www.migrainetrust.org

Offers information, advice and training to migraine sufferers and their families. Has a support network, funds research and runs conferences on migraine.

Other organisations

Benefits Enquiry Line

Tel: 0800 882200
Minicom: 0800 243355
Website: www.dwp.gov.uk
N. Ireland: 0800 220674

Government agency giving information and advice on sickness and disability benefits for people with disabilities and their carers.

British Association for Nutritional Therapy

27 Old Gloucester Street
London WC1N 3XX
Tel/fax: 0870 606 1284
Email: theadministrator@bant.org.uk
Website: www.bant.org.uk

Professional membership body for nutritional therapists. List of fully qualified practitioners available. Does not offer nutritional advice.

British Homeopathic Association

Hahnemann House, 29 Park Street West
Luton LU1 3BE
Tel: 0870 444 3950
Fax: 0870 444 3960
Email: info@trusthomeopathy.org
Website: www.trusthomeopathy.org

Professional body offering information about homoeopathy and list of accredited homoeopathic practitioners in local areas.

British Hypnotherapy Association

67 Upper Berkeley Street
London W1H 7QX
Tel: 020 7723 4443
Website: www.british-hypnotherapy-association.org

Professional organisation representing psychotherapists with at least four years of training in hypnotherapy. Provides full information about hypnotherapy and how it can help migraine sufferers. Can refer to nearest qualified therapist in your area.

British Medical Acupuncture Society

BMAS House, 3 Winnington Court
Northwich, Cheshire CW8 1AQ
Tel: 01606 786782
Fax: 01606 786783
Email: admin@medical-acupuncture.co.uk
Website: www.medical-acupuncture.co.uk

Professional body offering training in acupuncture to doctors, and list of accredited practitioners in local areas.

Chartered Society of Physiotherapy

14 Bedford Row
London WC1R 4ED
Tel: 020 7306 6666
Fax: 020 7306 6611
Email: csp@csp.org.uk
Website: www.csp.org.uk

Has information about all aspects of physiotherapy. Offers list of registered physiotherapists around the country.

General Chiropractic Council

44 Wicklow Street
London WC1X 9HL
Tel: 020 7713 5155
Fax: 020 7713 5844
Helpline: 0845 601 1796
Email: enquiries@gcc-uk.org
Website: www.gcc-uk.org

Professional body for chiropractors that can provide details of registered practitioners in your area.

General Osteopathic Council

Osteopathy House, 176 Tower Bridge Road
London SE1 3LU
Tel: 020 7357 6655
Fax: 020 7357 0011
Email: info@osteopathy.org.uk
Website: www.osteopathy.org.uk

Professional body for osteopaths that can provide
details of registered practitioners in your area.

NHS Direct

Tel: 0845 4647 (24 hours, 365 days a year)
Textphone: 0845 606 4647
Website: www.nhsdirect.nhs.uk
NHS Scotland: 0800 224488

Offers confidential health-care advice, information and
referral service. A good first port of call for any health
advice.

NHS Smoking Helpline

Tel: 0800 169 0169 (7am–11pm, 365 days a year)
Website: www.givingupsmoking.co.uk
Pregnancy smoking helpline: 0800 169 9169
(12 noon–9pm, 365 days a year)

Has advice, help and encouragement on giving up
smoking. Specialist advisers available to offer on-going
support to those who genuinely are trying to give up
smoking. Can refer to local branches.

National Institute for Health and Clinical Excellence (NICE)

MidCity Place, 71 High Holborn
London WC1V 6NA
Tel: 020 7067 5800
Fax: 020 7067 5801
Email: nice@nice.nhs.uk
Website: www.nice.org.uk

Provides national guidance on the promotion of good health and the prevention and treatment of ill-health. Patient information leaflets are available for each piece of guidance issued.

National Institute of Medical Herbalists (NIMH)

Elm House, 54 Mary Arches Street
Exeter EX4 3BA
Tel: 01392 426022
Fax: 01392 498963
Email: nimh@ukexeter.freeserve.co.uk
Website: www.nimh.org.uk

Professional body representing qualified practising medical herbalists. Offers list of accredited practitioners in the UK. An SAE requested.

OUCH (UK)

c/o Errington Langer & Pinner
Pyramid House, 956 High Street
London N12 9RX
Tel: 0161 272 1702 (24-hour answerphone)
Email: info@ouchuk.org
Website: www.ouchuk.org

Charity currently run almost solely by volunteers; their website offers the opportunity for members to exchange information on the chatline. Expects to set up support groups locally. Advice available via email and helpline.

Prodigy Website

Sowerby Centre for Health Informatics at Newcastle (SCHIN), Bede House, All Saints Business Centre
Newcastle upon Tyne NE1 2ES
Tel: 0191 243 6100
Fax: 0191 243 6101
Email: prodigy-enquiries@schin.co.uk
Website: www.prodigy.nhs.uk

A website mainly for GPs giving information for patients listed by disease plus named self-help organisations.

Quit (Smoking Quitlines)

211 Old Street
London EC1V 9NR
Tel: 020 72511551
Fax: 020 72511661
Helpline: 0800 002200 (9am–9pm, 365 days a year)
Email: info@quit.org.uk
Website: www.quit.org.uk
Scotland: 0800 848484
Wales: 0800 169 0169 (NHS)

Offers individual advice on giving up smoking in English and Asian languages. Talks to schools on smoking and pregnancy and can refer to local support groups. Runs training courses for professionals.

Society of Teachers of the Alexander Technique

1st Floor, Linton House, 39–51 Highgate Road
London NW5 1RS
Tel: 020 7482 5135
Fax: 020 7482 5435
Helpline: 0845 230 7828
Email: office@stat.org.uk
Website: www.stat.org.uk

Offers general information and lists of teachers of the Alexander technique in the UK and worldwide as well as recommended training schools. Members receive up-to-date information.

Websites

www.bash.org.uk
British Association for the Study of Headache (BASH)

UK national society, member of the International Headache Society (IHS). Membership is open to all health-care professionals with an interest in headache. The recently updated BASH Management Guidelines can be downloaded from the website.

www.migraine-disability.net/about_midas/about09.asp
MIDAS questionnaire

www.i-h-s.org
International Headache Society
Email: carol.taylor@i-h-s.org

Professional body for those involved in clinical or research work into headaches. Can put people in touch with local support groups.

www.w-h-a.org
World Headache Alliance
Email: carol.taylor@w-h-a.org

An international umbrella organisation to a number of global headache societies that can provide information on national groups. It has links to other relevant websites.

The internet as a further source of information

After reading this book, you may feel that you would like further information on the subject. The internet is of course an excellent place to look and there are many websites with useful information about medical disorders, related charities and support groups.

For those who do not have a computer at home some bars and cafes offer facilities for accessing the internet. These are listed in the Yellow Pages under 'Internet Bars and Cafes' and 'Internet Providers'. Your local library offers a similar facility and has staff to help you find the information that you need.

It should always be remembered, however, that the internet is unregulated and anyone is free to set up a website and add information to it. Many websites offer impartial advice and information that has been compiled and checked by qualified medical professionals. Some, on the other hand, are run by commercial organisations with the purpose of promoting their own products. Others still are run by pressure groups, some of which will provide carefully assessed and accurate information whereas others may be suggesting medications or treatments that are not supported by the medical and scientific community.

Unless you know the address of the website you want to visit – for example, www.familydoctor.co.uk – you may find the following guidelines useful when searching the internet for information.

Search engines and other searchable sites

Google (www.google.co.uk) is the most popular search engine used in the UK, followed by Yahoo! (http://uk.yahoo.com) and MSN (www.msn.co.uk). Also popular are the search engine provided by Internet Service Providers such as Tiscali and other sites such as the BBC site (www.bbc.co.uk).

In addition to the search engines that index the whole web, there are also medical sites with search facilities, which act almost like mini-search engines, but cover only medical topics or even a particular area of medicine. Again, it is wise to look at who is responsible for compiling the information offered to ensure that it is impartial and medically accurate. The NHS Direct site (www.nhsdirect.nhs.uk) is an example of a searchable medical site.

Links to many British medical charities can be found at the Association of Medical Research Charities website (www.amrc.org.uk) and at Charity Choice (www.charitychoice.co.uk).

Search phrases

Be specific when entering a search phrase. Searching for information on 'cancer' will return results for many different types of cancer as well as on cancer in general. You may even find sites offering astrological information. More useful results will be returned by using search phrases such as 'lung cancer' and 'treatments for lung cancer'. Both Google and Yahoo! offer an advanced search option that includes the ability to search for the exact phrase, enclosing the search phrase in quotes, that is, 'treatments for lung cancer' will have the same effect. Limiting a search to an exact phrase reduces the number of results returned but it is best to refine a search to an exact match only if you are not getting useful results with a normal search. Adding 'UK' to your search term will bring up mainly British sites, so a good phrase might be 'lung cancer' UK (don't include UK within the quotes).

Always remember the internet is international and unregulated. It holds a wealth of valuable information but individual sites may be biased, out of date or just plain wrong. Family Doctor Publications accepts no responsibility for the content of links published in this series.

Index

Your pages

We have included the following pages because they may help you manage your illness or condition and its treatment.

Before an appointment with a health professional, it can be useful to write down a short list of questions of things that you do not understand, so that you can make sure that you do not forget anything.

Some of the sections may not be relevant to your circumstances.

We are always pleased to receive constructive criticism or suggestions about how to improve the books. You can contact us at:

Email: familydoctor@btinternet.com
Letter: Family Doctor Publications
         PO Box 4664
         Poole
         BH15 1NN

Thank you

Health-care contact details

Name:

Job title:

Place of work:

Tel:

Name:

Job title:

Place of work:

Tel:

Name:

Job title:

Place of work:

Tel:

Name:

Job title:

Place of work:

Tel:

Significant past health events – illnesses/ operations/investigations/treatments

Event	Month	Year	Age (at time)

Appointments for health care

Name:

Place:

Date:

Time:

Tel:

Name:

Place:

Date:

Time:

Tel:

Name:

Place:

Date:

Time:

Tel:

Name:

Place:

Date:

Time:

Tel:

Appointments for health care

Name:

Place:

Date:

Time:

Tel:

Name:

Place:

Date:

Time:

Tel:

Name:

Place:

Date:

Time:

Tel:

Name:

Place:

Date:

Time:

Tel:

Current medication(s) prescribed by your doctor

Medicine name:

Purpose:

Frequency & dose:

Start date:

End date:

Medicine name:

Purpose:

Frequency & dose:

Start date:

End date:

Medicine name:

Purpose:

Frequency & dose:

Start date:

End date:

Medicine name:

Purpose:

Frequency & dose:

Start date:

End date:

Other medicines/supplements you are taking, not prescribed by your doctor

Medicine/treatment:

Purpose:

Frequency & dose:

Start date:

End date:

Medicine/treatment:

Purpose:

Frequency & dose:

Start date:

End date:

Medicine/treatment:

Purpose:

Frequency & dose:

Start date:

End date:

Medicine/treatment:

Purpose:

Frequency & dose:

Start date:

End date:

Questions to ask at appointments
(Note: do bear in mind that doctors work under great time pressure, so long lists may not be helpful for either of you)

Questions to ask at appointments
(Note: do bear in mind that doctors work under great time pressure, so long lists may not be helpful for either of you)

Notes

Notes

Notes